THE
BETTER LIFE
DIET©

*How to Live
a
Long and Youthful Life*

Second Edition

LESTER R. SAUVAGE, MD

of
The Hope Heart Institute
Seattle, Washington

with the assistance of
Robert H. Knopp, MD,
Northwest Lipid Research Clinic
University of Washington, and
Evette Hackman, PhD, RD and **Anna Ma**
of Seattle Pacific University.

cover by Arthur Nakata
illustrations by Warren
Berry and Kathryn Barker

also with
Carol Garzona, Linda
Plumb, and Stan Emert.

Better Life Press
Seattle, Washington

Publisher's Cataloging-in-Publication Data
(Provided by Quality Books, Inc.)

Sauvage, Lester R., 1926-
Better life diet and exercise program for a long and
       youthful life / Lester R. Sauvage. -- 2nd ed.
  p. cm.
    Includes index
    LCCN
    ISBN 0-9663788-4-9

    1. Nutrition. 2. Longevity--Nutritional
   aspects. 3. Exercise 4. Fitness   I. Title

RA784.S28 2001   613.2
                    QBI00-23

The Better Life Diet©
How to live a long and youthful life

TABLE OF CONTENTS

* This Appendix is a series of easily understood mini-lectures of key subjects pertinent to the matters addressed in this book. Reading this Appendix first may give you the broader insight needed to better appreciate the information and suggestions presented in Sections I-V.

Foreword by
Robert H. Knopp, MD
Professor of Medicine,
Director of the Northwest Lipid Research Clinic,
University of Washington

The public's interest in diets to lose weight without effort has never been greater. Dedicated scientists seldom have the opportunity to comment on the veracity of new dietary "discoveries" before they are enthusiastically reported in the media. Often fanned by conflicting claims, many diet books have become best sellers.

How can we explain the unquenchable desire of so many people for this information? My personal view is that changes in the American lifestyle, the lack of time to cook or even of families to eat together, and the penetration of public consciousness with advertising to consume convenient and not necessarily nutritious food-stuffs have left us in a state of progressive nutritional disorientation over the past 40 years. It is no wonder that people today are reaching out for help.

Consider the earlier situation. Typically women did the cooking. Skills were passed on to daughters who shared in the household responsibilities. Styles of cooking were governed by tradition and an agrarian history that favored preparation of a variety of homegrown fruits and vegetables, many of which were canned or frozen for winter. Sources of refined carbohydrates were fewer and were considered treats; highly sugared cereals didn't exist. Remember *Shredded Wheat?* By virtue of an agrarian or nearby agrarian tradition (like open air markets in cities) and without much premeditation, the right thing was being done for the most part with respect to fresh fruits, vegetables, and other unrefined carbohydrates.

The diet of those earlier days, however, was very rich in saturated fat. Perhaps the heavy farm work and industrial labor of yesterday made such foods less able to cause obesity and heart disease. But today our sedentary lives leave us unprotected. When frequent cigarette smoking was added in the 1900's, an explosive reaction occurred. Most hearts developed hardened coronary arteries. This led to the heart disease epidemic which Dr. Sauvage has spent decades combatting with his surgical knife and words of advice.

iv

Where are we now? In our modern life, healthy traditions are even more tenuous. Men and women are both responsible for the work of the home, including nutritional choices. But now, we rarely have heavy physical labor as a daily justification for a high-fat diet or as an antidote to obesity. Meanwhile, the TV so barrages us with ads trying to get us to buy foods we shouldn't eat that we become manipulated to try them. This conquest of mind and taste happens while we sit complacently in our chairs.

In finding new ways to eat well, the **Better Life Diet** that Dr. Sauvage espouses falls within the general boundaries of the sound nutritional and exercise recommendations offered by major national bodies, especially the latest (October 2000) iteration of the American Heart Association Dietary Guidelines. Dr. Sauvage studiously avoids extremism and takes advantage of the fact that restriction of saturated fatty acids, *trans* fatty acids, and total fats can lead to a reduction in blood cholesterol and body weight. With his recommended restriction of saturated and *trans* fatty acids to 10% or less of total calories, the fat intake from these threatening sources falls between the National Cholesterol Education Program's Step I and Step II Diets. Dr. Sauvage's program also avoids the high intake of refined carbohydrates and the blood sugar surges that ensue while providing essential fiber, antioxidants, and omega-3 fatty acids. The amount of protein he recommends is greater than that typically suggested but may aid satiety and spontaneous or intentional weight loss, in keeping with recent studies. The exercise that Dr. Sauvage recommends is both practical and essential to achieving normal weight and a sense of well-being. He properly emphasizes that both diet and exercise are necessary for a weight-control program to be successful. And this commitment must be for life!

Most importantly, this book is written with the intensity and directness of a leading heart surgeon and research director who draws on his extensive experience in repairing the ravages of advanced atherosclerosis and advising patients who know they are in trouble. In this age of fraying tradition, redistribution of responsibilities, media distraction, and jobs that provide no exercise, the **Better Life Diet** offers direct, no-nonsense, mainstream advice from a voice of great experience.

Preface

My objective is to help you live a long and youthful life through the wise application of dietary and exercise knowledge.

There are so many conflicting diets that the average person is left in a swirl of confusion. The *Pritikin* and *Ornish* diets advise about 80% of calories from carbohydrates, 10% from fats, and 10% from proteins. The *Atkins* diet advises almost no carbs initially while encouraging unlimited quantities of fats and proteins. The *Sugar Busters* diet avoids sugar. *The Omega Diet* focuses on types of fatty acids. The *American Heart Association* diet advises high-fiber carbohydrate intake with moderate fat restriction. The *Protein Power* and *Zone* diets advise high protein consumption.

I have selected the best from these diets and combined this information with what I have learned in taking care of thousands of patients, as well as advising many of their families and friends. As a heart surgeon I saw on a daily basis what disease can do to the heart. Clearly, **prevention** is the answer. For optimal results, diet and exercise must be combined into a unified program.

Most deaths from heart attacks, strokes, and limb loss; nearly all cases of lung cancer and emphysema; and most cases of adult-onset diabetes, blindness, and kidney failure can be prevented.

Is this possible? Yes, if you don't smoke, follow the **Better Life Diet and Exercise Program,** achieve and maintain a healthful weight, and control your psychological responses to life's challenges, *i.e.* stress! By making this lifestyle a reality, you will become empowered to attain the long and youthful life you desire. This is my goal for you!

Sincerely,

Lester R Sauvage

Section I:

Obesity

A Deadly but Curable Disorder

Obesity has become a major medical disorder that now causes millions of deaths worldwide each year. This disorder results from the storage of excessive quantities of fat in the cells of the adipose tissue. The main function of these adipocytes ("fat cells") is to store fat and regulate its distribution to the body's cells. Hundreds of pounds of excess fat can be stored in the adipocytes. In extreme cases, obese people become trapped in a sea of so much fat that they can barely move or breathe (Fig. 1).

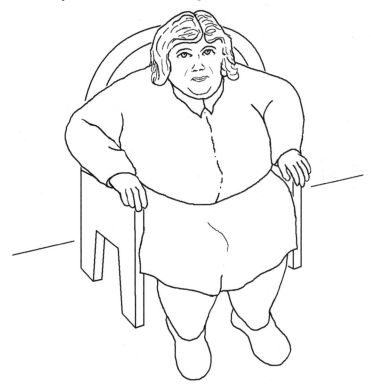

Figure 1 - Very obese woman, barely able to get up from her chair.

1

The adipose tissue is located just beneath the skin throughout the body (Figure 2). It is also present in the body cavities, more in the abdomen than in the chest.

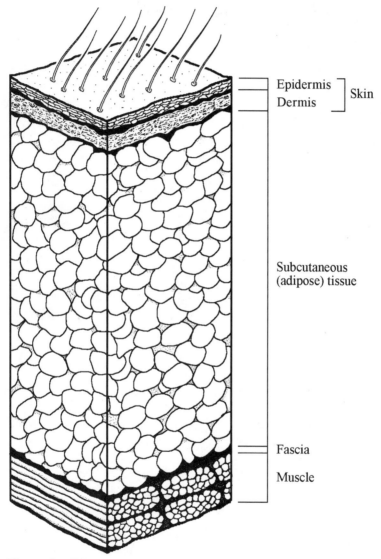

Figure 2 - Diagrammatic cross section of the skin, subcutaneous (adipose) tissue, and muscle in an obese person. Individual adipocytes in the globules of adipose tissue are not shown.

Obesity Kills

As the amount of fat in the adipocytes becomes excessive, increasingly serious medical consequences emerge. Obesity is an important cause of atherosclerosis (hardening of the arteries), which causes 95% of the deaths due to heart and artery diseases (heart attacks, strokes, and limb loss).

Obesity also causes about 90% of all cases of type 2 diabetes (p.81). In this type of diabetes the cells of the obese person lose their sensitivity to insulin* and cannot use sugar (glucose) properly for energy. As this loss of sensitivity develops, the islet cells of the pancreas try to compensate by secreting more insulin. This over-secretion hides the problem until the islet cells can no longer keep up, leaving the patient, now diabetic, resistant to what little insulin these exhausted cells can still produce. Diabetes is the most common cause of blindness and kidney failure. There are now 16 million diabetics in the U.S. and the number continues to rise.

In addition, obesity and type 2 diabetes are important causes of high blood pressure and congestive heart failure. But the good news is that both obesity and type 2 diabetes are disorders that can be largely prevented or corrected by a good diet combined with appropriate exercise. In the interest of our nation's health, we must resolve to act on this information.

A Worldwide Epidemic

There are now as many people in the world who are obese as there are people who are starving. Both obesity and starvation are deadly, but curable, conditions. Obesity is an advanced

* Insulin - A hormone secreted by the beta cells of the islets of the pancreas in response to the level of glucose (sugar) in the blood (pp. 81,84,85). This hormone enables the body's cells to use glucose for energy.

degree of being overweight. In the United States alone, 60% of people are overweight. Of these, *nearly half* (about 30% of all people) are obese (slightly more women than men). The obesity rate for Hispanic women is even higher, and for African-American women it approaches 50%.

Causes

Obesity is the result of a combination of eating too much, exercising too little, and having a genetic susceptibility to this disorder. The resulting state of excess fat storage can no longer be viewed simply as an unimportant condition. It's far more than a mere cosmetic state. Instead, obesity must now be regarded as a major abnormality because it threatens human health worldwide. Fortunately, of its three causes, the first two are correctable *and* preventable. For this reason, I believe that this deadly disease will be conquered through the power of enhanced education rather than by the magic of a much anticipated pill that may never be developed.

Obesity and Starvation are a Matter of Calories

Consuming too many calories makes us obese and consuming too few makes us gaunt and malnourished. Both of these conditions can kill. We want the healthy middle ground for ourselves and every living being.

Body fat in proper amounts is not a poison. Quite the contrary, fat is a vital component of every cell in the body. For example, the membranes surrounding all cells and their nuclei are formed of fat. In addition, 60% of the substance of the brain is formed from fat. Furthermore, fat is an important source of energy for the body.

Thus, fat stored in the adipocytes serves as an essential source for the fatty materials needed to maintain the structure and function of cells throughout the body, and to provide for reserve energy. Stored fat also serves two important passive functions - padding and insulation. Without padding, our bones would protrude through the skin. Without insulation, we would freeze in cold weather. Obviously, our body structure needs considerable fat. In fact, the fat content of normal-weight men is 15-20% of their body weight; and of normal-weight women, it is 20-25%. Yes, this is normal!

Every chemical component of the body can be over- or under-dosed, and fat is no exception. *Safety is a matter of dosage.* The amount of fat stored in the cells of the adipose tissue reflects the individual's caloric balance, i.e., calories in vs. calories out. Our goal is the healthy mid-range where we are neither too fat nor too thin.

Adipocyte Fat Storage Changes to Meet Need

Of the 100 trillion cells that comprise our mature bodies, about 100 billion are the adipocytes of the adipose tissue. These cells get bigger or smaller depending on the body's caloric balance and resulting need to store more or less fat in them. As the adipocytes enlarge, the person becomes visibly fatter. When these cells become smaller, the person becomes thinner (Figure 3). In addition, obese children may develop *more* adipocytes than their normal-weight counterparts. Very obese adults may do this, too.

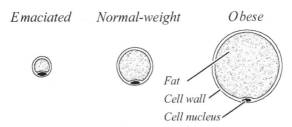

Figure 3 - Relative adipocyte size in emaciated, normal-weight, and obese people. Diet and exercise can reduce a big cell to normal size.

Apple- and Pear-Shaped Body Configurations

Obese men often store large amounts of fat in their abdomen, causing it to protrude and overhang their belts. This stored fat gives the abdomen an apple shape (Figure 4A). Because men with this shape have an increased risk of heart attacks, they have special need for preventive measures (pp. 13,14,16). Women, differing from men, often store large amounts of fat in their gluteal, hip, and thigh regions, which gives them a pear shape (Figure 4B). But women with this shape have the same risk of heart attacks as women who aren't overweight.

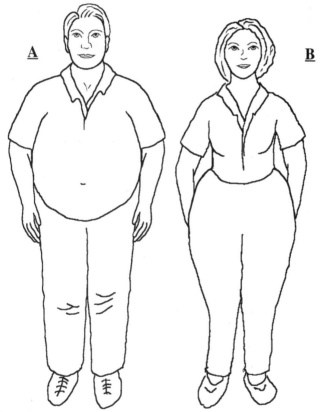

Figure 4 - (A) Apple-shaped accumulations of stored fat occur primarily in men. (B) Pear-shaped accumulations of stored fat occur primarily in women.

The Body-Mass Index (BMI)

General Considerations

The **Body-Mass Index** was developed to compare degrees of fatness in people. This index is a *relative* measure of the combined amounts of fat and muscle (protein) in the body.

People in the **healthy mid-BMI range** (Fig. 5, p. 8) maintain a sufficient, but not excessive, amount of stored fat to supply the body's needs for construction materials and energy without depleting their adipocytes. A proper diet and exercise program will keep you in this safe zone where you are neither too fat nor too thin and look and feel your best. This mid-range is where you want to be and want to stay.

People in the **high-BMI range** are *obese*. They have far more fat stored in their adipocytes than is safe (Figs. 1, 6, pp. 1, 9). This excess fat overflows the natural restraints and infiltrates the inner wall of many arteries, especially those of the heart (the coronary arteries). In addition, when the adipocytes become distended, cells throughout the body lose their sensitivity to insulin. Why this happens is unknown. The loss of sensitivity interferes with the normal use of glucose for energy and predisposes to the development of type 2 diabetes. This condition can set off an avalanche of illnesses.

People in the very **low-BMI range** are in a *starvation state*. Their caloric intake is so low they must burn their remaining fat for fuel (Fig. 3, p. 5). Then, these starving people burn their muscles for energy (Fig. 7, p. 11). In starvation, the body devours itself: carbohydrates first, fats second, and proteins (muscles) third. Starving people become so weak they can barely stand or even eat. They sleep and wait to die.

BMI and Normal Weight

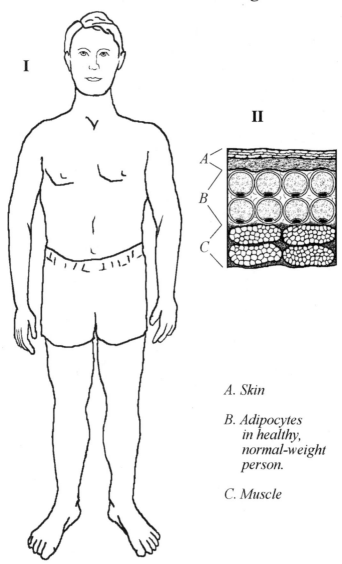

A. Skin

B. Adipocytes
   in healthy,
   normal-weight
   person.

C. Muscle

Figure 5 - (I) Normal-weight man in mid-range BMI category of 19-24 (see p. 10). (II) Diagrammatic cross section of skin, subcutaneous tissue, and muscle of this person. Adipocyte size and amount of fat stored in these cells is "normal."

BMI and Obesity

I   II

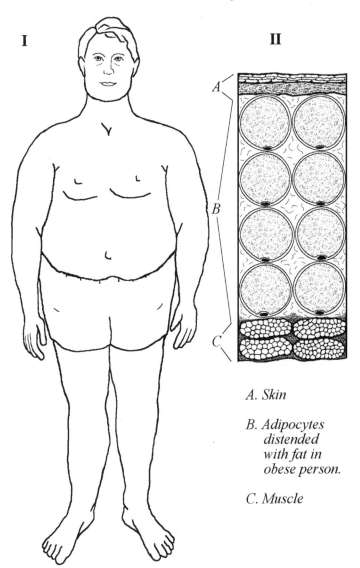

A. Skin

B. Adipocytes distended with fat in obese person.

C. Muscle

Figure 6 - (I) Obese man in high-range BMI category of 30 and above (see p. 10). (II) Diagrammatic cross section of the skin, subcutaneous tissue, and muscle of this person. Large increase in adipocyte size and amount of fat stored in these cells is apparent.

Specific Calculation Steps

The BMI can be simply estimated by multiplying the person's weight in pounds by 703 and dividing this result by their height in inches squared ($\frac{lbs. \times 703}{height\ inches^2}$). For example, if the individual is 5'10" (70") tall and weighs 176 lbs., the BMI calculated by this formula is 25 ($\frac{176 \times 703}{4900} = 25$).

Relation of Mid-BMI Range, and High- and Low-BMI Ranges to Bodily Health as shown in Figure 7, page 11

Healthy-weight people are in the *mid-BMI* range of 19-24 where their weight, muscle mass, and stored fat content proportions are proper. People in the elevated BMI range of 25-29 are considered overweight and have an increased body-fat content that is moderately dangerous to their health. People in the *high-BMI* range of 30 and above are classified as obese. They have such an increased amount of fat in their adipocytes (Fig. 3, p. 5) that it is a serious threat to their health. This danger worsens as the BMI increases. *At this point, please stop and calculate your own BMI. See where you are on both the fat and muscle parameters of Figure 7. Then calculate the pounds of fat you must lose or gain (p. 12) to get into the healthy mid-BMI range.* Short, broad-shouldered, muscular people score higher because of their specific body build.

People at the opposite end of the BMI scale (below 19) first develop a deficiency of body fat and then of muscle. This occurs as these tissues are sequentially consumed for fuel. Such people become emaciated as their BMIs fall to 15. At this BMI the fat stores are depleted and muscle is all that remains. The muscle must be burned rapidly to provide the energy to stay alive. This affects all muscles, including the heart. Starving people most often die from respiratory insufficiency when their muscles become too weak to support adequate ventilation. Pneumonia is often their final burden.

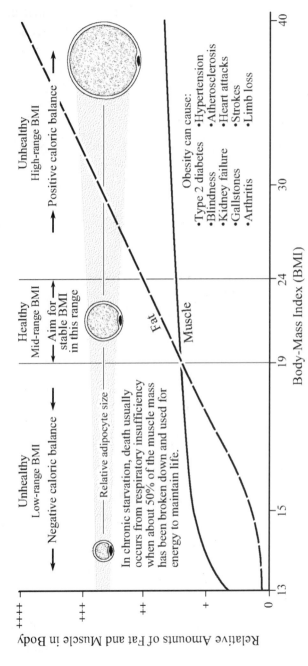

Continuum of BMI Relationship to Bodily Health

Unhealthy
Low-range BMI
← Negative caloric balance →

Healthy
Mid-range BMI
← Aim for →
stable BMI
in this range

Unhealthy
High-range BMI
← Positive caloric balance →

← Relative adipocyte size

In chronic starvation, death usually occurs from respiratory insufficiency when about 50% of the muscle mass has been broken down and used for energy to maintain life.

Fat

Muscle

Obesity can cause:
•Type 2 diabetes   •Hypertension
•Blindness   •Atherosclerosis
•Kidney failure   •Heart attacks
•Gallstones   •Strokes
•Arthritis   •Limb loss

Body-Mass Index (BMI)

13   15   19   24   30   40

Relative Amounts of Fat and Muscle in Body

0   +   ++   +++   ++++

Figure 7 - Shows the dynamic relationship of unhealthy low-, healthy mid-, and unhealthy high-BMI ranges to relative amounts of fat and muscle. [Caloric balance and adipocyte size relate only to the X (BMI) axis.]

Death from chronic starvation occurs when the BMI declines on average to 13. At that BMI, the body weight has decreased to about 1/2 of its "healthy" reading (Figs. 5, 7, pp. 8,11); the stored fat has fallen to about 5 to 10% of its "healthy" amount (Figs. 3,7, pp. 5,11); and the muscle mass has contracted to about 1/2 of its "healthy" volume (Fig. 7, p. 11).

Pounds of Fat an Obese or an Emaciated Person Must Lose or Gain to Get into the Healthy Mid-BMI Range

For a 236 lb. obese individual with a BMI of 32 and a height 6', I estimate the pounds this person needs to lose by adjusting the BMI formula as follows: 32 (current BMI) – 24 (target BMI) x $\frac{\text{height inches}^2 (5194)}{703}$ = 59 lbs. Thus, if this person loses a pound a week, he or she will require 59 weeks to get into the upper mid-BMI range. *Conversely, when fat is needed, lbs. required = target BMI – actual BMI x* $\frac{\text{height inches}^2}{703}$.

Caloric Balance Laws and the BMI

The basic facts cannot be changed. Eating adds calories; exercise uses them. We decide the balance. Apart from retaining water, we gain weight only when we take in more calories than we use *(positive caloric balance - law # 1)*. In a similar manner, we lose weight, apart from losing excess water, only when we use more calories than we take in *(negative caloric balance - law # 2)*. When we are in negative caloric balance, we burn stored fat to supply the difference. When the calories we eat equals the calories we use, our weight remains stationary *(isocaloric balance - law # 3)*. The BMI expresses these relationships.

These three laws mean that obesity can be conquered by diet and exercise. This wisdom needs support in the media. Instead, the most current *quick fixes* are "hyped" rather than presenting the basic truths that are needed to defeat this *deadly* disorder.

The Eight Principles That Make the
<u>Better Life Diet</u>
Obesity Correction Program Work

1. A consistently negative caloric balance (law #2) is necessary to lose the excess weight imposed by storage of too much fat in the adipocytes of the adipose tissue.

2. To lose excess stored fat, we must consume it for energy. There is no other way, short of surgery (p. 66), to eliminate excess fat. To burn a pound of stored fat/week requires a negative caloric balance of 600 calories/day. You can achieve this by decreasing your caloric intake (diet) and/or increasing your caloric output (exercise). This means that you must burn about 67 grams (9 cal./gram) or about $2\frac{3}{10}$ oz. of your excess stored fat everyday to supply these calories which your body is using in excess of the amount you are eating. To lose weight faster -- eat less, exercise more, or do both.

3. Proper weight loss is a slow process. In general, the faster off, the faster back. Crash diets seldom work because most people who try them relapse after initial success.

4. **A good daily exercise schedule is as essential to a successful obesity correction program as a good dietary plan is. Both are critical.** Exercise uses calories, increases the metabolic rate of the body, strengthens the heart and lungs, and builds the muscle mass which increases the body's *basal* metabolic rate. *Walking two miles briskly each day and lifting 3 to 6 lb. handweights in a deliberate, stretching (reach the sky) manner for five minutes morning and evening (p. 47) are excellent activities to attain these benefits.* This enjoyable combination of exercises can be done by nearly everyone.

5. Once you reach your mid-range target BMI weight (where you look and feel your best), you must continue your exercise

schedule and gradually increase your diet sufficiently to maintain this healthy weight *(but not more!)*.

6. *If you can get your weight down, you can keep it down.* The longer you remain at your target weight, the easier it becomes to stay there. This process resets your controls.

7. **Your diet and exercise program is for the rest of your life.** The *two main goals* of this program are for you to *lose your excess stored fat* and *increase your muscle mass.* Many stop their programs after they have lost several pounds. The result is predictable. Their weight rebounds, often to higher levels than before they started their programs. To prevent this from happening, *you must buy into the concept that your diet and exercise program is for life.*

8. To follow a diet and exercise program for life, your program must help you live each day in an invigorating manner. The five cardinal rules for healthy living comprise such a program (pp. 68-73). Try them. You'll become "fit" and be pleased.

The Essence of Weight Control

In summary, your weight is controlled by how much you *eat* and how much you *exercise.* By eating less and exercising more, you can achieve a negative caloric balance and *decrease* your *excess stored fat* while you *add muscle.* Obviously, a consistently negative caloric balance would, in time, prove fatal. The same is true of a consistently positive balance. If you are overweight, use a negative balance of 15-30% to get where you belong. Then level off and stay there.

When viewed in this context, the essence of weight control is simple. Practical application need not be difficult. The rest of this book provides the vital dietary and exercise information you need to live a healthy, fit, and happy life.

Section II:
Nutritional Basis for
The <u>Better Life Diet</u> and *Weight Control**

There are three basic types of foods: **carbohydrates (carbs), fats, and proteins.** Carbs and proteins are calorie poor (four calories/gram). Fats are calorie rich (nine/gram). Among other actions, carbs provide energy and fiber. Fats make cell walls, brain matter, hormones, and energy. Proteins form enzymes, antibodies, hormones, building materials, hemoglobin, muscles, and energy.

The **Standard American Diet ("S.A.D.") causes many to die prematurely.** It has too many calories, too many low-fiber carbohydrates (white bread, mashed potatoes, french fries, and white rice), far too much refined sugar, too much saturated fat, and too many *trans* fatty acids. *In addition to their improper and excessive diet, most Americans don't exercise nearly enough.*

Standard American Diet

1. Too many calories

2. Too much
- Low-fiber carbohydrates
- Refined sugar
- Saturated fats
- *Trans* fatty acids

3. Too little
- High-fiber carbs (vegetables, fruits, and whole grains)
- Legumes (peas, beans, and lentils)
- Mono and polyunsaturated fats (oils)
- Fish   • Nuts and seeds
- Nonfat/low-fat dairy products
- Skinless poultry
- Low-fat meat
- Shellfish

Figure 8 - Some deficiencies of the Standard American Diet.

* **We become what we eat. See the Appendix for discussions of atherosclerosis, carbohydrates, cholesterol, diabetes, fats, fiber, heart attacks, insulin, obesity, proteins, sugar, and *trans* fatty acids.**

Who doesn't look forward to sitting down with family and friends to enjoy a good meal? Though eating is pleasurable and necessary for life, we must control what we eat to live a long and healthy life. Our **Better Life Diet** does this. This diet is based on seven broad guidelines. It does not depend on detailed calorie counting. Enjoy this diet for life. Use it to lose or maintain weight as needed.

The Seven Guidelines of the Better Life Diet

To reduce obesity, adult-onset (type 2) diabetes, blindness, kidney failure, cancer, hypertension, atherosclerosis, heart attacks, strokes, and limb loss, we advise the following dietary rules:

1. **Eat plenty** of high-fiber carbohydrates, such as fresh fruits -- an apple a day is hard to beat; fresh vegetables; legumes (peas, beans, and lentils); whole-grain breads, cereals, and pastas; and whole grains, such as brown rice (p. 84).
2. **Markedly restrict** low-fiber carbohydrates, such as white bread, mashed potatoes, french fries, and white rice (p. 84).
3. **Drastically restrict** refined sugar, white or brown (p. 18).
4. **Choose** protective fats, i.e., oils (e.g., monounsaturated types, such as olive and canola, and polyunsaturated omega-3 types, such as fish and flaxseed -- pp. 81-83).
5. **Severely restrict** saturated fats and *trans* fatty acids (p.20).
6. **Enjoy** proteins with little saturated fat (fish; skinless poultry; eggs - p. 24; legumes; nuts; seeds; nonfat/low-fat dairy products; *low-fat meat*, as lean beef, lamb, and center cut pork loin/chop or roast; and *shellfish*, as clams, oysters, mussels, crabs, shrimp, lobsters, and scallops.
7. **Drink** at least two quarts of water a day (8 glasses).

If you are significantly overweight, this balanced diet of high-fiber carbs (50% of calories), protective fats (30%), and low-saturated fat proteins (20%), when combined with a good exercise program (pp. 13,14, 41-67), will autoregulate your weight over time to where you will feel and look your best and be able to stay that way.

Good Proteins - 20%
- Fish
- Skinless Poultry
- Eggs
- Legumes
- Nuts and Seeds
- Nonfat/low-fat Dairy
- Low-fat Meat
- Shellfish

4 cal/gm

Protective Fats - 30%

- 2/3 or more from mono and polyunsaturated oils
- 1/3 or less from saturated fats and *trans* fatty acids

9 cal/gm

High-Fiber Carbohydrates - 50%

- Fresh Fruits
- Fresh Vegetables
- Legumes - - Peas, Beans, and Lentils
- Whole-Grain Breads, Cereals, and Pastas
- Whole Grains, such as Brown Rice, Whole Wheat, Oats, Barley, Bulgur, and Rye

4 cal/gm

*Figure 9 - Building Block Diagram of the 50-30-20 **Better Life Diet** reflects the origin of approximately 50% of calories from carbohydrates (mainly high-fiber varieties), about 30% from fats (mainly protective mono and omega-3 and -6 polyunsaturated types), and about 20% from proteins (mainly those categories that have little association with saturated fats). Also see pages 23,24.*

More people are dieting. Yet more people are obese! Why? Too many diets fail to distinguish between high, low, and non-fiber (sugar - p. 22) carbs; saturated (bad) and unsaturated (good) fats; and high- and low-bad fat protein sources. Bad fats; *trans* fatty acids; and *excesses* of low-fiber carbs, refined sugar, and proteins (which are converted into saturated fat) decrease the liver's ability to remove LDL cholesterol (pp. 80, 81) from the blood. High blood levels of this chemical cause heart attacks and strokes.

To reduce LDL cholesterol, one must exercise and restrict whole milk, cream, butter, and foods made with them, such as high-fat cheeses, rich ice creams, pies, and cakes; poultry skin; fatty red meats; low-fiber carbs; refined sugar; and commercially processed, hydrogenated foods (p. 20), such as most margarines, crackers, cookies, candies, chips, dips, doughnuts, and desserts.

The average American eats **150 lbs.** of refined sugar/year, yielding 760 calories/day -- 38% of the calories in a 2,000 calorie diet. Sugar (sucrose) contains no fiber, minerals, phytochemicals (from plants), or vitamins -- only calories. Soda pop and watered-down juice drinks are full of sugar -- 10 teaspoons in a popular cola (ten times the total sugar -- glucose -- in all the blood in your body).

Real people in the real world need the **enjoyable meal plan** of *The Better Life Diet* (pp 31-40). This diet provides about **50% of calories from carbs**, mainly from high-fiber varieties (few from low-fiber carbs or refined sugar); **30% from fats**, mainly protective (liquid) types (*i.e.* oils); and **20% from proteins**, mainly those with little associated saturated fat. This tasty, filling, healthful, and practical high-fiber diet makes eating a pleasure, not a punishment.

Fiber, the portion of carbohydrates that our bodies can't digest, *is good for us because it slows digestion, reduces insulin secretion, minimizes changes in blood sugar, and decreases appetite.* (Imagine the "hype" for a drug that had these attributes!)

Most carb calories should come from fruits, vegetables, legumes, and whole grains and their products (few from white bread, mashed potatoes, fries, white rice, and refined sugar) - (pp. 16,17).

Most fat calories should come from oils, *i.e.* liquid (unsaturated) fats. Monounsaturated oils, such as olive, canola, avocado, and peanut oils are good for us. Some polyunsaturated oils are excellent, too, such as fish, flaxseed, and walnut oils (see p. 82 for omega-3 guidelines). Calories from saturated fats and *trans* fatty acids should not exceed 10% of the total calories you consume in a day. Saturated fats (such as butter) and hydrogenated oils (such as in many margarines) are soft solids at room temperature (p. 20). Excesses of these "hard" fats are far worse for our arteries than is enjoying a second egg for breakfast.

Most protein calories should come from fish (p. 24), *skinless* poultry; eggs; legumes; nuts; seeds; nonfat/low-fat dairy products; low-fat meat, such as lean beef, lamb, and center cut pork loin/chop or roast; and shellfish (p. 16). Few protein calories should come from *unskinned* poultry or *expensive* cuts of red meat (e.g., filet mignon) since both have a high content of saturated fat.

This high-fiber carbohydrate, unsaturated fat (oil), and low-sat.-fat protein **Better Life Diet** protects our arteries from hardening and clotting. This diet prevents marked rises and falls in blood sugar and related insulin secretion that cause recurring waves of profound fatigue, uncontrollable hunger, and excessive eating, all of which lead to obesity, type 2 diabetes, and hypertension - powerful risk factors for coronary heart disease (p. 81).

The **Better Life Diet combined with enjoyable daily exercise** (pp. 13,14, 47) is optimal for the vast majority of people who wish to look and feel their best. For the few whose livers can't remove LDL cholesterol from their blood (a "gene" problem, p. 77), we advise physician-prescribed cholesterol-lowering medications in addition to our **Better Life Diet and Exercise Program**.

Foods High in Saturated Fats
and
Foods High in *Trans* Fatty Acids

Restrict calories from saturated fats and *trans* fatty acids to not more than 10% of total calories consumed daily.

Saturated Fats:
1. Whole and even reduced-fat milk (p. 21), and foods made with these types of milk, such as high-fat cheeses.
2. Cream (sour/table/whipped), and foods made with cream, including rich ice creams.
3. Butter and foods made with butter.
4. Poultry skin (contains most of the fat in poultry).
5. Fatty (marbled) red meats.
6. Canned meats.
7. Processed meats such as bacon, lunchmeats (e.g., bologna, pastrami, and salami), and sausage.
8. Lard and foods made with lard.
9. Coconut, palm, and palm kernel oils, and foods made with these saturated tropical oils.

Trans Fatty Acids:*
1. Vegetable shortenings and foods made with them.
2. Many margarines and foods made with them.
3. Commercially processed foods made with hydrogenated "oils"* such as crackers, cookies, cakes, candies, chips, dips, doughnuts, pies, and other pastries.

---

* Many types of margarines and most commercially processed foods (as listed) contain hydrogenated soybean or other oils. Hydrogenation changes these oils into soft solids at room temperature. This change occurs because hydrogen is added to the molecular structure of the oils, and this produces *trans* fatty acids. Unfortunately, these acids are as dangerous as saturated fats because they also impede the removal of LDL cholesterol from the blood by the liver. This effect of hydrogenation causes the LDL cholesterol levels to rise. Such elevations become dangerous when they reach 130 mg/dL (an average value) -- pp. 80,81,87.

The **Better Life Diet** uses only nonfat or low-fat milk. There are four designations of milk according to its fat content: whole, reduced-fat, low-fat, and nonfat. Whole milk contains too much saturated fat and so does reduced-fat milk. A cup (8 ounces) of whole milk has 150 calories and 5 grams of saturated fat (4%); a cup of reduced-fat milk has 120 calories and 3 grams of saturated fat (2%); a cup of low-fat milk has 100 calories and 1.5 grams of saturated fat (1%); and a cup of nonfat milk has 80 calories and no fat. People who are lactose-intolerant can usually digest four ounces of milk at a meal or can drink calcium-fortified soy milk.

The areas of the **Better Life Diet** Building Block Diagram (Fig. 9, p. 17) accurately reflect the origin of calories from carbs (50% - 4 cal/gm), fats (30% - 9 cal/gm), and proteins (20% - 4 cal/gm). For a 2,000 calorie daily intake, this means 250 grams of carbs, 67 grams of fat, and 100 grams of protein.

The **Better Life Diet** emphasizes high-fiber carbohydrates, unsaturated fats (oils), and good proteins (Fig. 9, p. 17). While this diet doesn't eliminate any foods, it markedly restricts low-fiber carbohydrates (such as, white bread, mashed potatoes, french fries, and white rice), drastically restricts refined sugar (white or brown), and severely restricts saturated fats and *trans* fatty acids.

This tasty diet assures an adequate supply of calories (energy), building materials, fiber, minerals, phytochemicals, vitamins, and water. Also, the **Better Life Diet** markedly reduces the sugar stimulus for excess insulin secretion which further protects against obesity, type 2 diabetes, blindness, kidney failure, high blood pressure, atherosclerosis, heart attacks, strokes, and limb loss.

The **Better Life Diet** provides 30% of total calories from fat, mainly from unsaturated liquid types, such as olive, canola, nut, soybean, fish, and flaxseed oils. Even though these oils protect our arteries, they, like all fats, are so high in calories (9 calories/gram) that they must be taken in moderation. The **Better Life Diet** also requires a marked reduction in low-fiber carbohydrates and a drastic reduction in refined sugar (pp. 18, 84, 85 and below*).

We can learn much about the influence of diet on health from

----

* **Sucrose (table sugar) is digested rapidly. This drives the blood *glucose* up, which suppresses hunger and *causes the pancreas to secrete insulin*. Glucose falls. Hunger returns. When more sugar is eaten, the cycle repeats. *Fats and proteins have little effect on insulin.* Vegetables (because of their high fiber content) and fruits (because of their fiber and type of sugar -- fructose) convert more slowly into glucose and stimulate less insulin secretion. Milk sugar (lactose) causes a lesser insulin response, too. Insulin enables all the cells of the body to use glucose for energy, causes some excess glucose to be stored as glycogen (pp. 80, 84, 85), converts the remaining excess glucose into fat when the limited glycogen stores are filled (p. 28), and prevents fat from being used for energy.**

The up-and-down sugar-insulin relation fans the appetite; fats and proteins suppress it. Eating sugar throughout the day increases the secretion of insulin and enhances the manufacture of saturated fat from glucose, thereby negating the benefit of reducing the intake of saturated fat in the diet. But, markedly restricting low-fiber carbohydrates and drastically restricting refined sugar in the diet lowers insulin secretion and enables fat to be used for energy when the glycogen stores are exhausted. Making this source of energy available serves to help correct obesity and to prevent type 2 (adult-onset) diabetes, blindness, kidney failure, hardened arteries, hypertension, heart attacks, strokes, and limb loss.

The Better Life Diet *all but deletes* table sugar, standard soft drinks (soda pop), sugary "juice" drinks with less than 50% "fruit juice", jams, jellies, cakes, candies, pies, pastries, ice creams, and most other desserts. By following the Better Life Diet, the average daily consumption of refined sugar in a 2,000 calorie diet can be easily reduced from about 760 calories to 80 calories or less (pp. 31-40).

studies of **select population groups**. For example:

> **Japanese emigrants** to the U.S. who adopt our low-fiber carbohydrate, high-refined sugar, high-saturated fat, and high-*trans* fatty acid Western diet are at higher risk to develop obesity, type 2 diabetes, coronary heart disease, and breast and colon cancer than native Japanese living in Japan who eat their traditional high-fiber carb, low-refined sugar, low-saturated fat, and low-*trans* fatty acid native diet.

> Deaths from breast and colon cancer are uncommon in **countries where the diet is low in saturated (animal) fat.**

> **Seventh-Day Adventists** in the U.S. who restrict or avoid tobacco and meat have much less coronary heart disease, lung cancer, and emphysema than the general population.

The Five Basic Food Groups

Comparable Caloric Servings for the Different Food Groups

Fruits
- 1 whole medium-sized fruit like an apple, pear, or peach (about 1 cup - 8 oz.)
- 1/4 cup dried fruit
- 1/2 cup canned fruit
- 1/2 to 3/4 cup unsweetened fruit juice

Vegetables & Legumes

- 1/2 cup cooked vegetables or legumes
- 1/2 cup raw chopped vegetables
- 1 cup raw leafy vegetables
- 1/2 to 3/4 cup vegetable juice

Breads, Cereals & Pastas (whole grain)

- 1 slice bread
- 1 medium muffin
- 1/2 small bagel or English muffin
- 4 small crackers
- 1 small tortilla
- 1/2 cup cooked cereal
- 1/2 cup cooked rice
- 1/2 cup cooked pasta

Milk & Milk Products

- 1 cup (8 oz.) low-fat milk or yogurt
- 1 slice low-fat cheddar cheese, 1/8" thick (1 oz.)
- 1 cup of low-fat cottage cheese

Meat & Meat Alternatives

- 3 oz. (size of a deck of cards) cooked *lean* meat, skinless poultry, or fish*
- 2 eggs**
- 7 oz. tofu
- 1 cup cooked legumes (dried beans or peas)
- 1/2 cup nuts or seeds
- 2 tablespoons (32 grams - a little more than 1 oz.) of natural peanut butter - **not hydrogenated**

---

* **The omega-3 oils in fatty, cold-water fish, especially salmon, tuna, sardines, and trout, are protective of your arteries. Next to flaxseed oil, fish oil contains the largest quantity of these valuable polyunsaturated fatty acids. Eat fish frequently (p. 82).**

** **One to two eggs per day are good for you unless you are diabetic or have high blood values for LDL cholesterol and/or triglycerides. In that case we recommend that you limit eggs to 3 - 4/week. The liver makes about 3000 mg. of cholesterol/day. One egg contains about 200 mg. of cholesterol.**

How Many Servings Do **You** Need Each Day of the Five Basic Food Groups?

Calorie Level[1]	Children, Women, Older Adults	Teen Girls, Active Women, Most Men	Teen Boys, Active Men*
	About 1,600	About 2,200	About 2,800
Fruit Group	2	3	4
Vegetable and Legume Group	3	4	5
Bread, Cereal & Pasta Group	6	9	11
Milk & Milk Products Group[2]	2 to 4	3 to 5	4 to 6
Meat & Meat Alternatives Group	2	3	4
Grams of fat[3]	53	73	93

* Girls and women of comparable size, muscle mass, and activity level need the same number of calories as their male counterparts.

1. **Servings of the major food groups** required at different calorie levels for the **Better Life Diet** (pp. 16, 17).

2. **Teens, young adults, pregnant women, nursing women, and women concerned about preventing osteoporosis** need the higher number of servings (or additional calcium from alternative sources).

3. **Number of grams of fat when 30% of daily calories are from fat sources.**

20 Ways to Lower
the Saturated Fat and *Trans* Fatty Acid
Content of Your Diet

1. Microwave, bake, broil (on rack), poach, braise, or stir-fry foods instead of pan or griddle frying them when possible.

2. Use nonstick olive or canola cooking spray and a nonstick frying pan instead of adding butter or margarine.

3. Cook bacon and other fatty breakfast meats well, and then press them firmly between absorbent paper towels to remove as much of the remaining fat as possible.

4. Buy red meat with the least fat. "Prime" grade has the most fat, "choice" less, and "select" still less.

5. Purchase hamburger that is labeled "extra lean" and cook it well under the broiler to remove even more saturated fat.

6. Trim away all visible fat from meat before cooking and eating. This step can remove hundreds of calories.

7. Reduce the amount of saturated fat in canned meats, broths, and stews by chilling the cans before opening them. This causes the fat to rise to the top and solidify, making it easy to skim off.

8. Prepare foods in which the fat cooks into the liquid (stews, boiled meats, and soup stock) a day ahead of time. Then chill the food and remove the saturated fat which rises to the top and hardens.

9. Broil meats on a rack rather than frying them because the juices and liquified fat will collect in the pan below.

10. Defat these drippings if you make gravy with them by adding ice cubes to the drippings. This causes the fat to solidify and cling to the ice cubes, enabling it to be easily removed.

11. Limit meat to three 3-ounce servings (size of a deck of cards) of lean varieties a week. Eat more fish, poultry (without skin), eggs (p. 24), legumes (peas, beans and lentils), nuts, seeds, nonfat/low-fat dairy foods, and shellfish (pp. 16, 17).

12. Remove the skin before cooking poultry because most of the fat is in, or just under, the skin.

13. Eat turkey year-round, not just on Thanksgiving Day. The white meat eaten without the skin is best. It's lowest in fat.

14. Substitute mustard, ketchup, relish, mayonnaise, or salsa for butter or margarine in sandwiches.

15. Enjoy low-fat yogurt or nonfat sour cream on potatoes instead of butter or magarine.

16. Choose canola oil for low- or high-heat cooking but olive oil only for the lower-heat ranges. Both are protective of our arteries. In addition, olive oil is especially good for salads and bread dipping. Flaxseed oil also protects our arteries. Though excellent for salads, this oil is too heat-sensitive for cooking.

17. Switch from whole milk or reduced-fat milk to low-fat or nonfat milk. Your taste preference will change in several weeks. Once you've become accustomed to nonfat milk, whole milk will taste unbearably thick and fatty.

18. Remember that an "imitation" product may have as much or more "bad" fat as the natural product if it is based on hydrogenated and/or tropical oils. Read the labels.

19. Pick the softer margarines because they have fewer *trans* fatty acids. Squeezable margarines have the least, tub types intermediate amounts, and stick margarines have the most of these "bad" fatty acids (pp. 20, 71, 87).

20. Select low-saturated fat ("light," "diet," or "part-nonfat") cheeses and salad dressings instead of the high-fat varieties.

Basics for Weight Control

While the body can store little extra carbohydrate or protein, it can store almost limitless quantities of fat in the cells of the adipose tissue. *All digestible carbohydrates are converted into glucose.* Glucose stimulates the pancreas to secrete insulin, which rapidly converts any excess glucose (that not needed for energy and unable to be stored as glycogen) into saturated fat. Less than a pound of glycogen can be stored in the entire body, 1/3 in the liver and 2/3 in the muscles. High insulin levels block the use of fat for energy. As a result, a one way street is created -- fat in, no fat out.

But if low-fiber carbohydrates are markedly restricted and refined sugar is drastically reduced, weight reduction becomes relatively easy for most people - - if combined with a consistent, sensible exercise program (pp. 13, 14, 41-67). This dietary restriction reduces the insulin level in the blood and enables the excess fat stores to be used for the energy needs of the body (p. 22). At the same time, exercise increases energy needs and speeds fat loss (p. 65). The **Better Life Diet and Exercise Program** is also well-suited for people with Syndrome X (p. 87).

The **Better Life Diet** provides a balanced intake of carbs, about **50%** of calories (mainly high-fiber varieties), fats, about **30%** (mostly unsaturated -- liquid -- types), and proteins, approximately **20%** (mainly those with little associated saturated fat) to supply the energy, building materials, fiber, minerals, phytochemicals, vitamins, and water needed by our bodies. If you need to lose weight, eat less and exercise more; if your weight is satisfactory, continue as you are; and if you need to gain weight, eat more.

The building block diagram of the **Better Life Diet** on page 17 is a guide for developing such a balanced diet. The number of servings that you require of each of the main food groups depends on the extent of your caloric needs (p. 25).

Achieving and Maintaining Your Ideal Weight

Each person has an "ideal" weight that is best for his or her physiological makeup. When you follow the **Better Life Diet and Exercise Program**, your body will self-regulate over weeks to months (depending on need) to your proper weight range (Fig. 7, p. 11) and remain there so long as you stay with the program.

Nearly one in three Americans are obese. Obesity (excessive accumulation of fat) makes the heart work harder, predisposes to adult-onset diabetes, and produces biochemical changes that cause arteries to harden and wear out. Even losing only a few pounds of excess fat and *keeping these pounds off is important.*

People become overweight because they eat too much and don't exercise enough. **Losing this excess fat and adding muscle** requires a new way of living built around eating the right foods in the proper amounts and exercising *every* day (pp. 13,14, 41-67).

Crash diets *aren't* the answer. In the almost inevitable relapses that follow such diets, much more fat is added than muscle. The result is a fatter and weaker person who wonders what went wrong.

Weight Loss Strategy

If you are overweight, there is a pleasant solution for your problem: *start the* **Better Life Diet and Exercise Program**. Over the next month you will develop a taste for the diet (pp. 16, 17, 31-40), attain a full capacity for the exercise routine (2 miles of brisk walking daily and 5 minutes of slow, repetitive lifting 3 - 6 lb. handweights each a.m. and p.m.), and lose about 1 lb./week. If you wish to lose faster, increase your walking over the next month to four miles daily and don't eat *any* low-fiber carbs or refined sugar while adhering to the rest of your dietary and exercise plan.

On this accelerated program you will lose 1/2 to 1 pound *more* per week. When you reach your target weight, continue the **Better Life Diet** (pp. 16, 73, and Fig. 9, p. 17) **and Exercise Program** (pp. 13, 14, 46, 47, 54, 55, 70-72) at a level where you will look and feel your best indefinitely.

Excess weight is saturated fat waiting to be used for energy. The *two basic requirements* to begin the fat burning process are:
1. Consume fewer calories than you use (law # 2, p. 12).
2. Decrease your insulin secretion by severely restricting the low-fiber carbs and refined sugar in your diet. Reducing insulin secretion enables you to use your fat stores for energy (pp. 16,17, 22, 28, 85).

Combining these two dietary strategies with a good exercise program adds muscle and burns the excess stored fat.

Weight Gain Strategy
In the U.S., far more people need to lose rather than gain weight. But being very thin is dangerous, too. Emaciated people have minimal stored fat. If they become ill and unable to eat, they must burn their muscles for energy. Such people have no reserves and their immune systems become rapidly depleted.

If you need to gain a significant amount of weight, calories are what count. Eat four, five, or even six meals a day that appeal to your taste. If this approach doesn't work, contact your physician promptly. Unexplained weight loss needs to be investigated.

A note about alcohol: High consumption harms the heart, brain, and liver of both men and women. But in moderation, alcohol may have some protective action against coronary heart disease. Women are more sensitive to alcohol than men. Even in moderation, alcohol intake in women is associated with some increased risk of breast cancer. The reason for this is unknown.

Section III:

Seven day Meal Plan
for <u>The Better Life Diet</u>©
with Nutritional Analysis

Anna Martin and *Evette M. Hackman*, Ph.D., R.D.,
Department of Consumer Science, Seattle Pacific University

Some comments about following The Better Life Diet menu:

• Eating well should progressively become a way of life for you. Your body and mind will respond positively to the changes you are making. Please note, however, that fiber intake should be increased gradually in order to avoid the unpleasant side effects of a sudden "fiber overload," for example: gas, bloating, and abdominal cramping.

• As you look at the nutrition information for each day, you can see that eating is not an exact science. There will be some variation in your daily food intake and calorie distribution. Your goal should be to meet The Better Life Diet's 50/30/20 caloric percentages for carbohydrates, fats, and proteins, respectively, by the week's end rather than on a daily basis. Also, this meal plan has been constructed for a 2000 calorie diet. Your needs may be smaller or larger (p. 25).

• Under the daily nutrition information, the total sugar count includes naturally occurring sugars (found in fruits, some vegetables, and milk -- p. 22) as well as added refined sugar. For each day of the menu, the refined sugar comprises no more than 10% of the total sugar count. Also, for each day of the menu, the combined saturated fatty acids (SFAs) and *trans* fatty acids (TFAs) comprise no more than 10% of the total calories.

• Nuts & Nut Butters: Nutritionally, the best nuts to choose are peanuts, almonds, and walnuts, but do not feel restricted to these choices. When shopping for natural nut butters, look at the ingredient list. Peanut butter, for example, should read peanuts and salt only. Other varieties of nut butters are available at natural food stores, including cashew, hazelnut, macadamia, soy "nut", and more.

• **These menus were designed as guidelines to help you learn how to eat well and enjoy! Please view them as examples rather than the rule.** Here are some other valuable resources to help you on your way:

    1. *The Art of Nutritional Cooking, 2nd edition* by Michael Baskette and Eleanor Mainella. Upper Saddle River, NJ: Prentice-Hall, Inc.; 1999.

    2. *Sunset Quick, Light, and Healthy* by the editors of Sunset Books. Menlo Park, CA: Sunset Publishing Corporation;1996.

    3. *Cooking Light Magazine* by Doug Crichton, editor. Learn more on the web at www.cookinglight.com.

• Throughout the menu, when no beverage is specified, you may choose to enjoy *water*, coffee, tea, diet soda, or other **non-caloric** drink.

B = breakfast   **L** = lunch   **Sn** = snack   **D** = dinner

DAY 1 (vegetarian)

B: French Toast
> 2 pieces wheat berry bread
> 2 whole eggs
> cinnamon to taste
> topped with:
> > 2 teaspoons (tsp.) butter (about 8 grams)
> > 1/2 cup fresh berries (4 oz.)
> 1/2 cup fruit juice
> 1 cup (8 oz.) nonfat light yogurt

L: Garden Burger
> 1 vegetable burger
> 1 whole grain hamburger bun topped with:
> > 1 tsp. each: catsup, honey mustard, mayonnaise
> > 1/2 oz. reduced fat cheese
> > 2-3 slices of tomato
> > 2-3 leaves of spinach
> 1 oz. blue corn tortilla chips
> 1/4 cup salsa
> 1 cup nonfat milk

Sn: Fruit Smoothie
> 3 oz. soft tofu
> 1/2 mango
> 1/2 banana, frozen
> 1/2 cup guava nectar
> 1 packet Equal® sweetener
> 2 tablespoons (Tbsp.) nuts of choice

> **The Better Life Diet meets the nutritional needs for the vast majority of Americans in a tasteful, satisfying, and healthy manner (pp. 16-19).**

D: Curried Lentil Soup
> 1 cup (8 oz.) water with vegetable broth added
> 1/2 cup dry lentils
> 1/8 cup each: diced potato, carrot, celery, onion
> 1/8 tsp. each: ginger, garlic, curry powder
> 1 1/2 tsp. olive oil
> 1 medium slice wheat loaf bread oven-baked with
> > 1/2 oz. reduced fat cheese, shredded
> 1 cup spiced coffee (add dash of cinnamon & nutmeg before brewing)
> 1 small almond biscotti, 3-inch size

Nutrition Information: Day 1
Total Cal: 2043; % Carb: 53, % Fat: 28, % Pro: 19, SFAs+TFAs: 8.7%;
   Total Fiber: 46 grams (g); Total Sugars: 100 g (≤ 10% is refined).

DAY 2

B: Cold Cereal
1 cup Cheerios®
1/2 cup nonfat milk
1 banana, sliced
1/2 cup nonfat cottage cheese topped with
1 Tbsp. (about 1/2 oz.) each: raisins, sunflower seeds
1 cup fruit juice

L: Fish Soft Taco
2 oz. halibut dipped in lime juice and bread crumbs, then broil
cabbage slaw: 1/2 cup cabbage, 2 tsp. mayonnaise, pepper & rice
vinegar to taste
1 large garlic & herb flavored tortilla
2 Tbsp. salsa
fresh cilantro to taste
1/2 cup egg drop soup
8 oz. nonfat light yogurt
2 persimmons

> **The Better Life Diet supplies all the daily requirements for vitamins and minerals.* (pp. 39, 40)**

Sn: Hummus with Pita
1/2 wheat pita pocket, cut into 4 wedges
top each wedge with:
2 Tbsp. hummus
1 each: tomato slice, cucumber slice, fresh mint leaf

D: Grilled Vegetable & Ham Sandwich
1 medium sized whole wheat hoagie roll
1 oz. ham, deli meat
1 cup grilled vegetables: eggplant, squash, tomatoes, mushrooms,
bell peppers
1 oz. Havarti cheese spread on roll:
1 Tbsp. plain nonfat yogurt
1/2 tsp. Dijon mustard
1-2 cloves roasted garlic
1 tsp. olive oil (about 1/6 oz.)
1/2 cup nonfat cottage cheese
1 cup watermelon slush, blend together:
1 cup watermelon cubes, frozen
1 packet Equal® sweetener
1 1/2 Tbsp. lemonade, frozen concentrate

Nutrition Information: Day 2
Total Cal: 1983; % Carb: 53, % Fat: 26, % Pro: 22, SFAs+TFAs: 6%;
Total Fiber: 36 g; Total Sugars: 143 g (≤ 10% is refined).

* For additional protection, we advise selected supplements (pp. 42,75).

DAY 3

B: Vegetable Omelet
>   2 whole eggs
>   1 cup diced vegetables: tomatoes, bell peppers, mushrooms,
>   onions
>   1/2 oz. reduced fat cheese
>   2 Tbsp. salsa
>   2 pieces whole wheat toast topped with
>   2 oz. herbed yogurt cheese*
>   1 orange

L: Quick & Easy Bagel
>   1 whole wheat bagel, halved and toasted, topped with:
>   2 Tbsp. natural peanut butter
>   1 banana, sliced
>   1 cup nonfat milk

Sn: Trail Mix
>   1/2 cup Wheat Chex® cereal
>   1/4 cup assorted dry fruit
>   2 Tbsp. nuts/seeds of choice
>   8 oz. nonfat light yogurt

> **People who need less than 2,000 calories a day, especially women, should maintain a high milk, yogurt, and cheese intake to provide necessary calcium.**

D: Salmon
>   3 oz. salmon fillet
>   marinate in 1/4 cup soy sauce, fresh ginger & garlic to
>   taste, then bake
>   1/2 cup steamed asparagus tips
>   topped with 1 tsp. butter
>   1/2 yam, sliced and oven grilled
>   topped with 1 tsp. butter
>   2/3 cup nonfat, sugar free ice cream topped with:
>   1/4 cup fresh berries
>   2 Tbsp. chopped nuts of choice

Nutrition Information: Day 3
Total Cal: 2078; % Carb: 53, % Fat: 27, % Pro: 20, SFAs+TFAs: 7%;
     Total Fiber: 45 g; Total Sugars: 100 g (≤ 10% is refined).

*Note: Yogurt cheese can easily be made by straining plain yogurt overnight in the refrigerator through either a very fine mesh strainer or cheesecloth. Discard the liquid portion and season the cheese as desired (i.e.: sun-dried tomatoes, onion and dill, roasted garlic and thyme - - be imaginative).

DAY 4

B: Breakfast Sandwich
1 whole wheat English muffin, toasted
1 whole egg, fried with non-stick spray
2 pieces turkey bacon
1/2 oz. reduced fat cheese
1 orange
1 cup nonfat milk

L: Quick Three Bean Chili
1 Lean Cuisine Three Bean Chili® entree
1/2 oz. reduced fat cheese
2 tsp. light sour cream
1 piece jalapeño corn bread, from mix
topped with 1 tsp butter
1 cup watermelon
1 cup nonfat milk

> The Better Life Diet provides
> healthy food with great taste
> for a long life.

Sn: Filled Tortilla
1/4 cup cooked black beans
1/8 cup cooked brown rice
1 oz. reduced fat cheese
2 Tbsp. salsa
1 whole wheat tortilla filled, folded, and fried in 1 tsp olive oil
2 tsp. light sour cream

D: Pork Kabob
marinade: 1/2 cup apple juice, 1 Tbsp olive oil, cloves, garlic, herbs
marinate the following, then skewer with 2 bamboo spears & grill:
2 oz. pork tenderloin, cubed
1/2 cup potato, cubed
1/2 cup asparagus tips
1/2 apple, cubed
4 pearl onions
1/2 cup cooked brown & wild rice
1 cup nonfat milk
1 Dole® fruit juice bar

Nutrition Information: Day 4
Total Cal: 2010; % Carb: 50, % Fat: 28, % Pro: 22, SFAs+TFAs: 10%;
Total Fiber: 35 g; Total Sugars: 91 g (≤ 10% is refined).

DAY 5

B: Oatmeal
    1 cup cooked oatmeal stir in:
        2 Tbsp. natural peanut butter
        1 packet Equal® sweetener
1 apple
1 cup nonfat milk

L: Turkey Sandwich
    2 pieces rye bread
    1 oz. skinless turkey breast
    top with:

> **The Better Life Diet provides delicious food at low cost.**

        1/2 oz. reduced fat cheese
        1/4 of an avocado
        1 tsp. Dijon mustard
        spinach, tomato, red onion, black olives to taste
2 kiwi
1 cup nonfat milk

Sn: English Muffin Pizza
    1 whole wheat English muffin, toasted
    top each half with:
        2 Tbsp. spaghetti sauce
        1/2 vegetarian sausage link, sliced
        1/4 oz. reduced fat cheese

D: Peanut Chicken Stir Fry
    3 oz. skinless chicken breast
    1 cup stir fried vegetables (snap peas, bell pepper, zucchini,
        carrots, broccoli, mushrooms)
    1 cup brown rice
    peanut sauce - heat in saucepan then pour over stir fry dish:
        2 Tbsp. each: Teriyaki sauce, natural peanut butter
        1/4 tsp. each: fresh chopped ginger, crushed red pepper chili
            flakes
        1 tsp. sesame oil
1 fortune cookie
1 cup Lipton® spiced chai tea, made with equal parts nonfat milk and
    water
1 packet Equal® sweetener

Nutrition Information: Day 5
Total Cal: 2038; % Carb: 50, % Fat: 29, % Pro: 21, SFAs+TFAs: 6.1%;
    Total Fiber: 45 g; Total Sugars: 88.6 g (≤ 10% is refined).

DAY 6

B: Breakfast Shake & Bagel
>1/2 banana, frozen
>1/2 cup each: frozen strawberries, orange juice, lowfat buttermilk
>1/2 tsp. each: vanilla extract, nutmeg

1/2 whole wheat bagel
1 Tbsp. almond butter

L: Pita Sandwich & Soup
>1/2 wheat pita pocket stuffed with:
>>2 oz. skinless chicken breast
>>fresh spinach & artichoke hearts
>>1 oz. feta cheese
>>red pepper pureé, blend together and spread inside pita:
>>>2 oz. water packed roasted red pepper
>>>2 tsp. olive oil
>>>1 tsp. each: fresh parsley, capers, minced garlic

1 Nile Spice® Instant Minestrone cup of soup
1 orange
1 cup nonfat milk

Sn: Tuna & Crackers
>1/4 cup water-packed tuna mixed with:
>>2 Tbsp. chopped celery
>>2 tsp. mayonnaise

8 Triscuits®
1 apple

> **Crash diets aren't the answer.
> The *Better Life Diet and
> Exercise Program* is the
> answer (pp. 28-30).**

D: Spaghetti With Meat Sauce
>1 cup vegetable sauce with:
>>1/2 cup tomatoes
>>1/4 cup each: zucchini, mushrooms
>>Italian spices to taste
>>1 tsp. olive oil
>2 oz. extra lean ground beef
>1 1/2 cup whole wheat spaghetti noodles
>top pasta dish with
>>1 Tbsp each: pine nuts, parmesan cheese

1/2 baked pear

Nutrition Information: Day 6
Total Cal: 2012; % Carb: 53, % Fat: 28, % Pro: 19, SFAs+TFAs: 7.4%;
>Total Fiber: 42 g; Total Sugars: 98 g (≤ 10 % is refined).

DAY 7 (fast food)

B: McDonald's
> 1/2 Apple Bran Muffin
> 1 serving pork sausage
> 1 carton orange juice
> 1 carton milk, 1 % *

L: Wendy's
> Grilled Chicken Sandwich
> Deluxe Garden Salad, nonfat dressing
> 1 apple**
> 1 carton milk, 2 % *

Sn: Muffin & Yogurt
> 1/2 Apple Bran Muffin (from breakfast)
> 8 oz. nonfat light yogurt**
> 1 small box raisins**
> 1/2 cup baby carrots**

D: Pizza Hut
> 2 pieces Veggie Lover's® pizza
> 1 orange**

> **Combine the Better Life Diet with two miles of continuous brisk walking and ten minutes of slowly lifting 3 to 6 lb. handweights every day (pp. 13, 14, 46, 47, 54, 55).**

Nutrition Information: Day 7
Total Cal: 1894; % Carb: 51, % Fat: 30, % Pro: 19, SFAs+TFAs: 10%;
   Total Fiber: 20.3 g; Total sugars: 128 g ($\leq$ 10% is refined).

* Nonfat milk would be best. The milk designated, however, is the type that was sold at these fast food restaurants in the Seattle area at the time we wrote these sample meal plans.

** Indicates items that must be brought from home.

Note: This menu was included as an example of how to enjoy a balanced meal on the occasions that you eat at a fast food restaurant. As you can see, you do not need to totally eliminate these foods from your diet. Most fast foods, however, tend to have excess amounts of low-fiber carbohydrates, refined sugar, saturated fats, *trans* fatty acids, calories, and sodium. In addition, your body often does not get enough fresh fruits and vegetables when you eat out frequently.

7 Day Averages
of
Nutrients, Vitamins, and Minerals
for
The Better Life Diet©
Sample Meal Plan Analysis

	7 day averages -	Percent of US Label Adult RDA

Basic Components

Calories	2008.56	97%
Calories from Fat	570.08	213%
Protein	106.55 g	91%
Carbohydrates	271.82 g	151%
Dietary Fiber	37.68 g	
Soluble Fiber	7.50 g	
Sugar - Total	107.84 g	
Monosaccharides	29.62 g	
Disaccharides	36.47 g	
Other Carbohydrates	102.46 g	97%
Fat - Total	63.34 g	85%
Saturated Fat	17.00 g	
Mono Fat	21.64 g	
Poly Fat	9.87 g	
Trans Fatty Acids	0.48 g	94%
Cholesterol	283.42 mg	
Water	1619.35 g	

Vitamins

Vitamin A (RE)	1587.21 (RE)	159%
A - Carotenoid	841.68 (RE)	
A - Retinol	340.02 (RE)	
A - Beta Carotene	4200.00 mcg	(700 RE)

RDA = Recommended Daily Allowance
g = gram
mg = milligram

mcg = microgram
RE = Retinol Equivalents

Thiamin-B1	1.66 mg	111%
Riboflavin-B2	1.99 mg	117%
Niacin-B3	21.06 mg	105%
Niacin Equivalent	33.25 mg	166%
Vitamin-B6	2.07 mg	103%
Vitamin-B12	3.72 mcg	109%*
Vitamin C	211.73 mg	353%
Vitamin D	5.51 mcg	55%
Vitamin E-alpha equiv.	9.71 mg	108%
Folate	341.33 mcg	85%
Pantothenic Acid	5.74 mg	57%

Minerals   Food Label Value *

Calcium	1451.68 mg	145%
Copper	1.52 mg	76%
Iron	16.94 mg	94%
Magnesium	366.93 mg	92%
Manganese	4.74 mg	100%
Phosphorus	1478.80 mg	148%
Potassium	3831.87 mg	109%
Selenium	99.21 mcg	150%
Sodium	2608.52 mg	109%
Zinc	9.40 mg	63%

Other Fats

Omega-6 Fatty Acids	7.03 g
Omega-3 Fatty Acids	0.69 g
	Ratio -10:1 **

Other

Alcohol	0.21 g
Caffeine	19.64 nanograms

** A ratio of 4:1 or less is better. Taking one teaspoon daily of pleasant tasting flaxseed oil (richest source of omega-3 fatty acids - 2100 mg/tsp) would reduce the ratio to 2.7:1. I take one teaspoon daily of Barleans Lignan Rich Flax Oil obtained from Barleans Organic Oils, 4936 Lake Terrell Road, Ferndale, WA 98248. Phone 1-800-445-3529.

Section IV:

Exercise - - Essential Ally of Diet

Diet without exercise is like a car with four flat tires. It can't go very far. This is why we emphasize that exercise is the essential ally of diet. But, exercise must be **aerobic** ("with oxygen") to benefit your body. Aerobic exercise *doesn't* deplete your muscles of oxygen, make you short of breath, or cause you to perspire heavily (unless it's very warm). On the other hand, **anaerobic** ("without oxygen") exercise *does* deplete your muscles of oxygen, make you breathless and unable to speak, and cause you to perspire heavily.

Anaerobic exercise demands more oxygen and nutrients than your arterial blood can deliver to your overworked muscles. It also produces more waste products than your blood can remove. Such excessive exercise makes you severely short of breath, causes your pulse to race, and wears you out quickly. It's neither safe nor good for the average non-athletic person.

Aerobic exercise, however, is performed at a pace which is within the capacity of your circulation to deliver the extra oxygen and nutrients that your working muscles need. Your blood also removes carbon dioxide and other waste products from your muscles. You can continue this rhythmic muscular activity for long periods with a stable, moderately elevated pulse rate without becoming breathless, exhausted, or drenched in sweat. Aerobic exercise is safe and good for you. Combine it with the **Better Life Diet** for health and happiness.

The ability to talk while exercising *(the talk test)* is a simple way to tell whether an exercise is "aerobic" for you. If you can carry on a normal conversation, it is; if you can't, it's anaerobic. People in poor shape fail the *test* while walking slowly; people in good shape pass while walking briskly; people in excellent shape pass while jogging. Regardless of the activity, adjust your pace so you can pass the "*test*."

Regular aerobic exercise:

- **Costs little in time or money.**
- **Uses calories.**
- **Increases joy in life.**
- **Tones and enlarges muscles.**
- **Sharpens your mind.**
- **Alleviates depression.**
- **Reduces stress.**

- **Promotes sound sleep.**
- **Strengthens heart and lungs.**
- **Lowers risk of osteoporosis.**
- **Assists the whole body to use oxygen and nutrients more efficiently.**
- **Helps the digestive system to work better.**
- **Improves dangerous blood chemistries.**

Regular weight-bearing aerobic exercise also helps women after menopause prevent or slow the development of osteoporosis, a process that absorbs bone structure and weakens the skeleton. The protective effect of exercise is enhanced by the *Better Life Diet* and by taking vitamin D, calcium, magnesium, and estrogen (or related compounds).

Severe osteoporosis weakens bones so much, especially of the hips and spine, that they break easily. This occurs more often in elderly women, but strikes men as they age, too. Even without obvious fractures of the backbone, osteoporosis silently shortens the spine of both men and women and causes them to lose height in their advancing years.

A few points need emphasis. We all need aerobic exercise to help strengthen bones, increase muscle size and power, lose excess stored fat (weight), improve heart and lung function, and gain a renewed sense of vigor. The benefits of aerobic exercise promote fitness and help prevent osteoporosis, obesity, type 2 diabetes, blindness, kidney failure, clots, hypertension, atherosclerosis, heart attacks, congestive heart failure, strokes, decreased walking capacity, and limb loss.

In brief, regular aerobic exercise is the closest thing we have to an **"anti-aging pill."** You'll find that life's a lot more fun when you take this "pill" every day.

Walking briskly without becoming winded is hard to beat as an exercise for many reasons. It's safe, pleasant, inexpensive, good for most everything, and able to be enjoyed nearly any time and any place. Try it! Two miles in the morning or evening will do wonders for you. This is a habit to form, combine with **The Better Life Diet,** and practice for life.

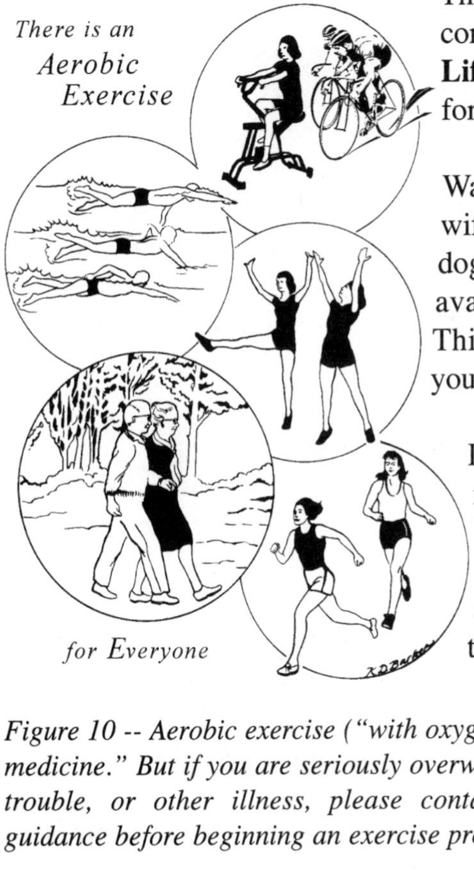

There is an Aerobic Exercise

Walk with your husband, wife, children, friend, or dog. If none of them are available, walk alone. This is time you owe yourself. Precious time.

If you can't walk two miles, try one. If not one, do what is comfortable for you and slowly increase the distance.

for Everyone

Figure 10 -- Aerobic exercise ("with oxygen") is good "every day medicine." But if you are seriously overweight, and/or have heart trouble, or other illness, please contact your physician for guidance before beginning an exercise program.

F.I.T.
The Basics:
Frequency ... Intensity ... Time

The first thing to know about "regular aerobic exercise" is that unless you do it *frequently enough, intensely enough,* and *long enough,* it's not going to do you, your cardiovascular, respiratory, or muscular systems, or your weight reduction program much good.

As an aid to getting in shape and staying that way, think F.I.T. for the **frequency**, **intensity**, and **time** of exercise.

Frequency

The American College of Sports Medicine recommends daily aerobic exercise to achieve fitness. I agree and believe that we need daily exercise just as much as we need to eat everyday. We need to use our muscles consistently to keep them and our heart and lungs in shape. There's no way around this requirement. *We either use our muscles or we lose them* -- an easy choice if we wish to get in shape and stay fit.

Intensity

Most of the mystique that surrounds aerobic exercise has to do with its intensity or "pace."

Take *"the talk test"* to find the aerobic pace that's right for you (pp. 41, 42). Increase your pace to where you can't carry a conversation and then slow down to where you can. Don't exercise on the "edge." You need some "breathing room."

When you're in the "groove," you'll work up a moderate

sweat, but you won't get breathless. If you find yourself huffing and puffing and unable to carry on a conversation, slow down and find the pace that's right for you. Leave long distance running and triathlon competition to the athletes. It's not healthy for you to go to the edge of your endurance. *A brisk two mile walk and lifting light handweights slowly for ten minutes each day are superb exercises.* You will find them easy to perform, enjoyable, and effective.

Time

Many studies show that we need at least 30 minutes of aerobic exercise most days of the week for reasonable fitness.

There is some controversy here, however. A panel of experts convened by the American College of Sports Medicine and the Centers for Disease Control (CDC) recently announced that *accumulating* 30 minutes of "moderate exercise" each day (e.g., walking, gardening, climbing several flights of stairs, and/or doing housework *every* day) is enough to improve overall fitness, at least moderately. Researchers at the Harvard School of Public Health believe, instead, that 45 minutes of daily, brisk, *continuous* exercise is preferable.

The bottom line is that even a *little* exercise is better than no exercise, and in general, *more* exercise is better than less exercise -- within reason of course.

Thirty minutes of daily aerobic exercise will help you attain and maintain your optimal weight. If you need to lose weight faster, perform 45 to 60 minutes of continuous aerobic exercise once or, if necessary, twice a day. This need not be complicated. Just go out, start walking, and build from there.

Questions and Answers
About Exercise

Q. *What are the different types of exercise?*

A. 1. **Isometric exercise** (muscle contraction without
motion) tones the tensed muscles, but uses few
calories.This type of exercise doesn't improve *overall*
cardiovascular, respiratory, or muscular fitness.

2. **Isotonic exercise** (muscle contraction with motion,
e.g. weight lifting) is far more valuable than isometric
exercise. Lifting heavy weights is not practical for
most middle-aged and older people. *But doing several
sets of lifting 3 to 6 lb. handweights slowly to the point
of some muscle fatigue daily is practical.* This simple
routine builds arm, shoulder, back, and pectoral
muscle size and strength. Increased muscle mass
raises your metabolic rate which burns more stored fat
even while you're resting (p. 65).

3. **Anaerobic exercise** *(without* adequate oxygen) -
- such as sprinting or fast cycling -- leads to
exhaustion and breathlessness in a few minutes.
Physical benefits can't be realized when the body is
running short of oxygen. Also, severe anaerobic
exercise can be dangerous for the non-trained person
because it quickly depletes the heart of oxygen.

4. **Aerobic exercises** *(with* adequate oxygen) such as
walking, dancing, jogging, golfing (preferably
without a cart), cycling, swimming, handball, tennis,
and rowing can be continued for long periods
without becoming breathless if your pace is right.
These exercises build muscle, get your heart and

lungs in shape, help you attain and maintain a healthful weight, and keep you in good condition. **This combination of benefits could save your life!**

Q. *Should I check with my doctor before beginning an exercise program?*

A. Yes, if you:
- Are 35 years of age, or older.
- Haven't seen your physician for over a year.
- Have a personal or family history of cardiovascular disease.
- Are a smoker, or have high blood pressure.
- Are seriously overweight.

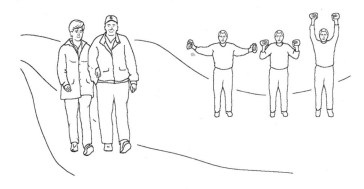

Special Note: It is important to find exercises that you *like* to do. There are many for you to choose from in this section. My favorites are those shown above. At age 74, I greatly enjoy briskly walking two miles each evening with my wife. Also, I enjoy lifting three-pound weights in a slow, repetitive, stretching (reach the sky) manner for five minutes each morning and evening. I am confident that this practical exercise routine, requiring about 45 minutes a day, could also help you enjoy a long and youthful life. *Be innovative in developing a program you will look forward to each day.*

Q. *How can I find time to exercise?*

A. The same way you find time every day to eat and sleep. Exercise is just as important. Make it a priority.

Q. *What are my exercise choices?*

A. There are many. The following comments about the more popular aerobic exercises are to pique your interest and get you involved.

1. Aerobics

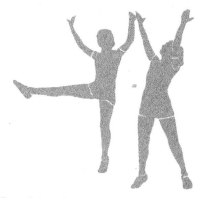

Special Advantages:

- Special fun for those who like exercising to music. Such music can sway your soul.
- Entire body is exercised.
- Group spirit is established in the classes.
- Necessary skill is rapidly acquired. Beginners become "pros" in a short time.
- Classes are held inside, away from the weather.
- Many styles of aerobics and different kinds of music to choose from.

Special Equipment and Facilities Needed:

- Loose-fitting clothing and comfortable shoes with cushioned soles (athletic shoes give the best support).
- Space and a qualified instructor.

Advice for Beginners:

- Talk to your friends and find out what program and which instructor they enjoy and why. If that doesn't work, check with the registered programs in your community, such as those at the YWCA or YMCA, and ask what they offer. Then talk to their instructors.

- Sign up for classes with a friend. You'll encourage each other and have lots of fun.

- The typical aerobic dance program consists of a one-hour class Monday, Wednesday, and Friday for three months. But some aerobics classes are only offered twice a week. Unfortunately, this schedule doesn't provide enough exercise to get your cardiovascular, respiratory, and muscular systems in good shape. To get more exercise, sign up for an additional program, or supplement your classes with other aerobic exercises that you do on your own, such as walking or swimming.

- Make sure you exercise strenuously enough in your class to work up a moderate sweat, but don't get so carried away that you become breathless and drenched in sweat.

2. Cycling

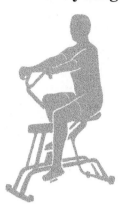

Special Advantages:

- Especially well-suited for older and overweight individuals, and for those with back, knee, and/or foot problems.

- Outdoor bikes can be used for transportation.

- Indoor bikes protect you from the weather and allow you to watch television while pedaling.

Special Equipment Needed:

- An outdoor or indoor bike. These may be purchased or rented from a cycle shop. Want ads and garage sales may be useful in finding a good second-hand bike.

- Before purchasing a bike, check consumer magazines, read a bicycle book, and talk with friends. If you still need more guidance, consult a fitness professional. Then comparison shop.

- Outdoor bikes should have at least three gears.

- Indoor bikes must have an adjustable tension control. All other special features are optional.

Advice for Beginners:

- Have a bike specialist "fit" your bike to your body by adjusting the seat and handle bar heights and positions so your legs and back are comfortable

- Outdoor cyclists should wear helmets because they provide needed protection against devastating head injuries in case of an accident.

- Work on finding a pedaling pace and tension control that will give you an adequate workout without causing shortness of breath. If you get to a point of breathlessness, slow down until you catch your breath. Then pick your pace up to the point you're sweating some but aren't winded.

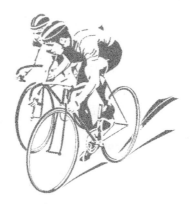

3. Swimming

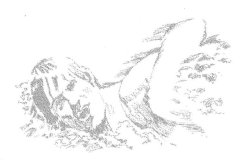

Special Advantages:

- Well-suited for most everyone who can swim and especially those with back and/or joint problems which restrict or prohibit them from enjoying other popular aerobic exercises.

- The perfect aerobic exercise for those who want a good workout but hate to sweat.

- Works on all body muscles.

Special Equipment and Facilities Needed:

- Swim suit.

- Eye and ear protection, if necessary.

- A swimming pool. Check out the pools operated by the parks department, YMCA, YWCA, and local health clubs. Be sure that the pool you select is large enough for nonstop lap swimming. You need space for this.

Advice for Beginners:

- Inquire when your pool opens and closes. Some run from 5:00 A.M. to 10:00 P.M. Avoid the crowded times. Even fish need room to swim.

- Use any stroke and get in as much nonstop lane swimming as possible during your exercise time. If you start to lose your breath, slow down. Once you've caught your breath, find your proper stroke and pace.

- If it's difficult for you to get to a pool on a regular basis, use the other suggested aerobic exercises to supplement your swimming program. In doing this, don't forget how important it is that your daily activity routine be enjoyable for you.

Swimming and Osteoporosis:

- Studies have shown that swimming *doesn't* strengthen your bones. If you're concerned about osteoporosis, get plenty of *weight-bearing* exercise, such as walking, which does strengthen your bones.

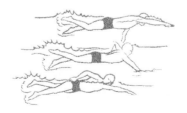

4. Walking

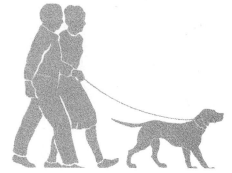

Special Advantages:

- This is the best exercise for the great majority of us because it's easily within our capabilities, is an enjoyable challenge to our bodies, and is a rich source of health benefits (pp. 42, 43).

- Two miles of brisk walking daily is a superb base for the exercise program of most people, young and not as young.

- Can be used for transportation.

- Provides the same benefits as jogging, with less risk of injury.

- No expertise needed; you've been doing it since you were one year old.

Special Equipment Needed:

- Comfortable shoes with cushioned soles that give you good, stable support - - that's all you need. You can't beat this for simplicity.

Advice for Beginners:

- If you're out of shape, begin slowly and first increase the distance and then your pace, but do this in a careful, progressive manner. If you become breathless or don't feel comfortable, you're going too fast . . . slow down! When you've caught your breath, continue at a pace that enables you to talk normally.

- Over a period of weeks to months, work up to a level where you can briskly walk nonstop for 30 to 60 minutes without feeling winded.

- Don't count the stop-and-go casual walking you do around the house or at the office as part of your walking program. Stop-and-go exercises don't provide enough conditioning benefits for your heart and lungs. Set special time aside for brisk, nonstop walking. These are precious moments *you owe yourself.*

- Overweight people find that the addition of nonstop, brisk walking to their daily routines can help them lose weight without having to severely reduce their caloric intake.

- When you reach a point where you need more of a challenge, strap on a weighted backpack or add a few hills to your walking program.

- Notes on brisk-walking form: Swing your arms, take long strides, and look at the beautiful world around you. Remember that you are an important part of this scene, too.

5. Jogging

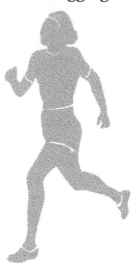

Special Advantages:

* Especially effective in increasing the secretion of a chemical (nitric oxide) by the endothelial cells that line the blood vessels. This causes the small arteries to enlarge and the blood flow to increase. Nitric oxide also makes the vessel lining smooth and slippery. These changes reduce clot and plaque formation.

* It's fun and motivating to jog with a companion if you like company during exercise. Pick a buddy, however, who's approximately at your level of fitness. If he or she is in much better shape, you will be run ragged. If your companion lags far behind in speed and/or stamina, you won't be able to get to the level of exercise that you need.

Special Equipment Needed:

- Quality running shoes (not sneakers) are essential to protect your feet and joints from the pounding they take in jogging. Shoes should extend 3/4" beyond the longest toe, fit perfectly over athletic socks, allow no slippage of the heel, be sufficiently flexible (even when new) to be comfortable, and have shock-absorbing soles.

- Hundreds of brands and varieties of running shoes are available. Shop around until you find a perfect fit. In general, athletic stores tend to have wider selections and more experienced salespeople.

- Dress in layers when it's cold; don't overdress when it's warm.

- If you have knee and/or foot problems, you may need to see an orthopedist or a podiatrist to obtain special instructions and/or an orthotic shoe insert.

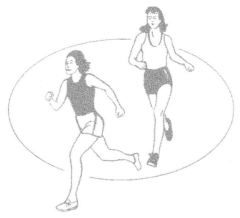

Beginning Jogging

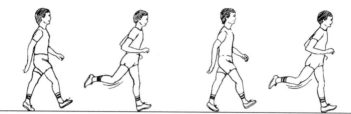

Alternate walking with slow jogging.

Advice for Beginners:

- Invest in a good book on jogging before beginning your program.

- At first, alternate walking with slow jogging, slowing to a walk whenever you reach the point where you can't talk normally. Gradually increase the proportion of jogging time to walking time until you are jogging on a nonstop basis. Don't expect too much too soon. You will get there. Be patient!

- If you feel you are able to do more, extend your time, not your speed (pace).

- Don't try to keep up with others who are in better shape than you. Exercise at your own pace. *You* are in charge!

- Take time to "warm up" and stretch. This is important to help prevent injuries.
- Stay within your improving exercise capacity.
- Don't lean forward when you jog.
- Hold your forearms approximately parallel to the ground, and keep your hands and shoulders relaxed.
- Keep your stride short -- don't let your feet get out ahead of your knees.
- Land on your heels, not on the balls of your feet. Sore feet are no fun.
- Breathe through your mouth.
- When you're within about 10 minutes of stopping your exercise session, slow your jogging pace down gradually *and finish by walking at a comfortable pace for several more minutes.* This allows time for your circulation to clear the lactic acid from your muscles in order to avoid having them become stiff and sore. Treat your muscles with respect.

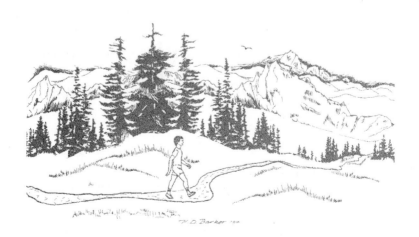

Times to Exercise

Before Breakfast

Advantages:

- Raises your metabolic rate early in the day.
- Clears your mind and invigorates your body so you can begin your day with enthusiasm.
- At this refreshing time of day, it's hard to make excuses for not exercising.
- You have to take a shower anyway.

Possible Disadvantages:

- It may be hard to get out of bed a little earlier.

Before Lunch

Advantages:

- Works off morning tensions.
- Refreshes you to meet the afternoon demands.
- Helps curb lunch appetite.

Possible Disadvantages:

- You may need to shower and not have an opportunity to do so.
- Your lunch break may not be long enough for you to complete an adequate exercise session and still have time to eat.

Before Dinner

Advantages:

- Clears away the day's worries.
- Refreshes you for evening activities.
- Helps curb dinner appetite.

Possible Disadvantages:

- Easy to find a reason not to exercise at this time of day.

After Dinner

Advantages:

- Clears your mind and helps you relax.
- Walking following eating helps your digestive system to work better and doesn't require waiting. (Both my wife and I like to take our evening walk shortly after we have cleared the dinner table and put the dishes in the dishwasher.)

Possible Disadvantages:

- Easy to say -- "It's late, I'll do it tomorrow."
- You may need to wait for an hour or more after you have eaten before doing certain types of exercise, such as jogging or calisthenics.

There are a million excuses for not exercising regularly. Here are a few:

"I don't have the time."

All it takes is a minimum of 30 minutes of aerobic exercise most days to stay in reasonable shape. You'll be set if you take 10 minutes from your usual TV watching time, 10 minutes from your sleep time, and 10 minutes from your goof-off time and use these minutes for vital aerobic exercise everyday. You can't lose with this trade-off - - a real bargain!

"I don't have the energy."

The vast majority of people who exercise regularly say exercise makes them "feel full of energy," and that's why they do it. Exercise, by getting the blood circulating and the muscles moving, is an ideal way to overcome frustration, relieve stress, and clear your mind of the day's problems. In this way, it serves to supply you with more energy, providing a kind of "second wind" that recharges your batteries.

"I always get sore."

Sore muscles result from doing too much, too soon, and not coming to a gradual stop. Start a routine where you gradually increase the time of exercising before increasing the speed (pace). Before stopping, slow down gradually over 5 to 10 minutes, so your muscles won't become stiff and sore (p. 59).

"It's too much work to get in shape."

A nice thing about aerobic exercise is that you can adjust the pace to suit your needs. You'll soon find the right speed that will allow you to progressively extend your exercise time to 30 minutes without becoming breathless.

"I've tried getting more exercise, but I never stick with it."

This time you will! You can afford 30 minutes of exercise on most days of the week. No big deal! If you need a motivator, exercise with a buddy, use gold stars on a calendar, or anything that works for you. The key is to *make exercise a high priority* and develop it into a faithful habit.

"I'm too old."

You're only as old as you feel and regular exercise makes you feel younger. Start slowly, and work on *gradually* increasing your muscular, cardiovascular, and respiratory endurances.

"I hate fighting the weather."

An indoor swimming pool, exercycle, shopping mall (for walking), or an aerobics class can help. If these don't suit your fancy, get a treadmill, and walk *inside* on rainy days.

"I have arthritis."

Your doctor may recommend that you cycle or swim indoors, or do both. Studies show that these exercises will help relieve your arthritic pains and stiffness and limber you up.

"I'm too busy running around doing things for other people."

In order to help others more effectively, you must first take care of yourself. A half-hour of aerobic exercise most days is a gift you *must* give yourself. It will allow you to feel and look your best, and enable you to do more for others.

"Exercise is boring!"

Well, see what you can do to make it "fun"! Vary your walking/jogging route. Listen to music. Position your indoor bike so you can watch the evening news while you pump away. Join an aerobic dance class. Exercise with a friend. Treat yourself to new athletic shoes. Challenge yourself.

"I don't know what to do with the kids."

If possible, take them with you (they need exercise, too!). There are walking/jogging strollers on the market made for children. One of these could enable your young son or daughter to enjoy the ride while you supply the power. And, many health clubs have child day-care facilities; check them out. You may also wish to pick up an indoor bike or treadmill.

"My family isn't interested."

That's okay. This is something you're doing for yourself.

"I'm not that interested in fitness; I've got other priorities."

Stop for a moment and reflect: "Exercise will help me live longer and better." And that's for real! And there's more.

Difficult problems often "solve themselves" while you exercise. This isn't an illusion. Exercise refreshes your mind and helps you think more clearly.

"I don't have the right clothes, equipment, etc."

Buy them. It could be one of the most valuable investments of your life. Why not? You owe this to yourself.

"I'm too fat."

So . . . you're just the one who needs to exercise. Start with something easy, like walking around the block. Do that for a week. Go around twice the next week, and so on. See how much better you'll feel -- and how much less you'll want to eat! Keep at it, and you'll begin to feel better and better as you progressively lose excess fat while you gain needed muscle. Don't forget that losing excess fat stores is just a matter of using more calories than you take in (caloric law # 2, p. 12).

"According to the charts, I'd have to jog forever just to work off one doughnut."

Exercise charts only tell half the story. First of all, many people find that regular aerobic exercise helps them curb their appetite. One reason for this is that exercise tends to reduce tension and depression, common causes of the "munchies." Exercise also signals the liver to convert some of its glycogen into glucose and release it into the blood, which helps curb the appetite.

Second, muscles which are exercised on a regular basis use more energy (calories) even when resting than muscles which have not been exercised. Exercise "tunes" the body's engines (muscles) so they idle faster at rest.

In addition, the muscles of people who exercise on a regular basis get bigger. As a consequence, fit people, pound per pound, burn more calories than fat people because a pound of resting muscle burns more calories than a pound of fat. This difference in caloric consumption becomes even more pronounced after exercising and lasts for many hours.

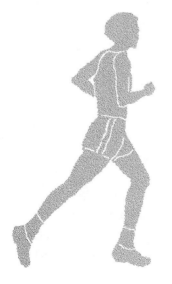

Have faith. If you have a large amount of fat to lose and are only losing one pound per week, don't get discouraged. You're on track. Fifty pounds in a year is a lot. Remember, the right way to lose weight permanently is to lose excess stored fat gradually while you add muscle (pp. 28-30).

"I will just exercise the fat parts of my body."

It's true that fat tends to concentrate in specific areas of the body. It generally shows up around the waists of men and in the hip and thigh regions of women (Fig. 4, p. 6).

Spot-reduction exercises like sit-ups and leg-lifts make the abdominal muscles stronger and firmer. The same fat deposits, however, still sit on top of those muscles. The fat on top of a muscle does not belong to that muscle; it belongs to the whole body. This fat will begin to "melt away" only when the demand for calories in the whole body exceeds the caloric intake. We keep coming back to this basic fact.

In general, spot-reduction exercises don't use as much energy as whole-body aerobic exercises, such as walking or jogging. These whole-body exercises are better because they use larger sets of muscles and require more calories to meet the increased energy requirements. And when you use more calories than you eat, you lose weight. Simple as that.

Remember, excess stored fat depresses the metabolic rate, while added muscle increases it. The more muscle you have, the more fat you will burn. This is so, provided you reduce your caloric intake and blood insulin level (p. 22) by severely restricting low-fiber carbohydrates and refined sugar.

Special Note: I advise plastic surgery for removal of fat deposits *only* when these deposits are very persistent and disfiguring. A currently popular operation for this purpose is called **liposuction**. In this procedure, the plastic surgeon inserts a tubular suction device through the skin and uses it to slim and contour the excessively padded areas by literally sucking out the adipose tissue. Though this technique is indicated for some patients, it's an **expensive and**

potentially dangerous way to lose fat. In most cases, there is a better way: *The Better Life Diet and Exercise Program!*

"I had coronary bypass surgery three weeks ago, and I don't know if it's safe for me to begin an exercise program."

If you are gaining strength, feeling better, and able to walk up a flight or two of stairs without becoming short of breath or developing chest pain, your doctor will be delighted! In fact, he or she will likely start you on a progressive walking program at that point.

Your physician will follow your progress closely. When you are ready, he or she will extend the distance you walk and, later, increase your pace. Your doctor may also refer you to a cardiac rehabilitation program near your home. There are good programs in most areas of the United States today. They promote proper diet, exercise, health education, and confidence.

Exercise is an important part of both your short-term and long-term treatment plans. Don't become impatient and go too fast early on, or become too busy to exercise later on.

Remember, the time you take to exercise is a precious gift you owe yourself and your loved ones. *Make your exercise and diet program a high priority* because it is vital for you to enjoy a long and youthful life in the years ahead.

Section V:

A Simple Plan
for a Long
and
Youthful Life

Preventable fatalities (p. 69) account for about 75% of all premature deaths in the US. Adherence to the *Five Cardinal Rules for Healthy (Fit) Living* will help you avoid most of these illnesses and extend your life.

General Considerations

Heart attack and stroke are the leading killers in the industrial world. But the good news is that the death rate for cardiovascular disease in the U.S. has decreased about 20% in recent years. But the rising incidence of obesity and type 2 diabetes threatens to reverse this favorable trend. There is still much for us to do.

Hardening of the arteries (atherosclerosis) begins early in life. *Autopsy examinations of adolescent American accident victims show that most already have fatty plaques in their coronary arteries.* These findings indicate that we must start in childhood to prevent heart disease from developing. This can be done by teaching today's children the rules of healthy, fit living in three interrelated ways:

1. Good example and instruction by parents in the home. This is vital!
2. Positive guidance by pediatricians and family physicians.
3. Proper training by teachers in the schools.

"An ounce of *prevention* in early years is worth a pound of *cure* in later years." But prevention efforts must be both *simple* and *effective* if they are to be widely adopted as a way of life.

Our guidelines pass this test. Simply said, they are: *don't smoke, closely follow the **Better Life Diet and Exercise Program**, attain and maintain a healthful weight, and control stress.*

These guidelines will help you avoid developing obesity, atherosclerosis, hypertension, clots, heart attacks, strokes, decreased walking capacity, limb loss, congestive heart failure, aneurysms, hemorrhages, many types of cancer (especially of the lung), emphysema, adult onset (type 2) diabetes, blindness, kidney failure, gallstones, and degenerative arthritis.

In addition, these guidelines are vital if you have had surgery for heart or artery disease. This is because surgery is only a *mechanical* solution to a structural problem. You also need to prevent the development of more atherosclerosis (pp. 78, 79).

Given enough time, all arteries will eventually wear out. In earlier years so many people died of infections (such as smallpox, pneumonia, influenza, typhoid, diphtheria, tuberculosis, staph infections, strep infections, meningitis, and appendicitis) that few lived long enough for this to happen. In fact, most people died before reaching age 50.

Now that we are living longer (the average life span in the U.S. is about 74 years for men and 79 for women), about *half* of us will die prematurely from hardened arteries and clots unless we take steps now to prevent this from happening later.

The Five Cardinal Rules
for
Healthy (Fit) Living

To increase our chances of living to a ripe old age with our mental faculties and physical capabilities in top form, it's necessary to follow an effective plan to keep our arteries in good condition. Our plan may be expressed through the following five letters: **S ... D E W ... S** which identify the core subjects of the five cardinal rules for healthy, fit living:

Smoking ... **D**iet-**E**xercise-**W**eight ... **S**tress.

Our prime objective is to prevent the development of atherosclerosis which causes clots to form that block the flow channels of vital arteries. The program works in two main ways. *First,* it lowers the blood levels of LDL cholesterol, triglycerides, glucose, and homocysteine while elevating those of HDL cholesterol and omega-3 fatty acids. *Second,* the program decreases the blood's ability to clot by lowering the level of fibrinogen and by keeping platelets from becoming too sticky. These actions keep blood flowing throughout our bodies. This is vital! **The five cardinal rules are:**

#1
_S_moking **Don't smoke**, or be around those who are smoking. This helps to prevent atherosclerosis, heart attacks, strokes, limb loss, cancer, and emphysema.

#2
_D_iet **Follow** the **Better Life Diet** (pp. 15-40), a meal plan consisting of high-fiber carbohydrates, protective fats, and good proteins. This diet severely restricts low-fiber carbohydrates, refined sugars, saturated fats, and *trans* fatty acids. It helps to prevent hypertension, atherosclerosis, heart attacks, strokes, limb loss, cancer, obesity, type 2 diabetes, blindness, kidney failure, gallstones, and degenerative arthritis. This healthy diet is also delicious. The engaging taste of its many foods makes eating a joy to anticipate and a pleasure to realize.

#3
_E_xercise **Perform** 45 minutes of **aerobic exercise** each day (pp. 41-67). Two miles of nonstop brisk walking daily and 5 minutes of repetitive lifting 3 to 6 lb. handweights in a slow, stretching (reach the sky) manner each A.M. and P.M. are hard exercises to beat.

#4
_W_eight **Attain and maintain** your **ideal weight**. This is the weight at which you feel and look your best.

#5
_S_tress **Strive** for the **inner peace** that allows you to willingly accept problems as a challenging part of life. You can best achieve this mental state free of harmful stress by traveling the road of God's *Golden Rule* to loving human relations.

The 5 Cardinal Rules for a Healthy (Fit) Lifestyle

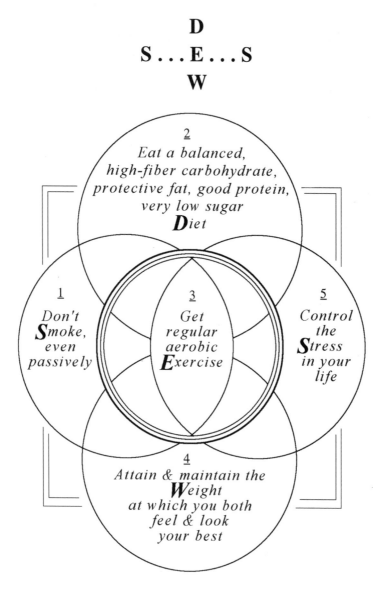

Figure 10 - The five interlocking rules for healthy living are vital for a long and youthful life (for diet, see p. 16 & Fig. 9, p.17).

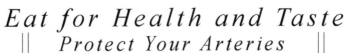

Eat for Health and Taste
Protect Your Arteries
& Enjoy Life

*Fresh fruits,
fresh vegetables,
& legumes*

*Fish &
poultry without skin*

Eggs, may have 1-2 per day*

Drink nonfat milk

*Whole grain breads, cereals,
& pastas*

*Markedly restrict low-fiber carbohydrates
(white bread, mashed potatoes,
french fries, & white rice)*

Drastically restrict refined sugar

*Severely restrict saturated fat,
and <u>trans</u> fatty acids*

** For people who don't have either diabetes or
elevated LDL cholesterol and/or triglycerides.
(For those who do, please see pp. 24 and 80-83)*

*Figure 11 -- **The Better Life Diet** --
Delicious foods that are good for you.*

Three Additional Strategies

If people would follow the five cardinal rules for healthy living, the incidence of heart attacks, strokes, limb loss, cancer, hypertension, obesity, type 2 diabetes, blindness, and kidney failure would decrease dramatically. But some need more. These are the people who have a family or personal history of heart or artery disease at a young age (35 - 40 years) or have one or more of the following threatening blood chemistries:

1. An HDL cholesterol level below 35 mg/dL in men and below 45 mg/dL in women. The higher this value the better because HDL transports LDL cholesterol out of the blood and the arterial wall.

2. A fasting blood glucose value above 120 mg/dL.

3. A fasting triglyceride level above 200 mg/dL. A value of under 100 is ideal. (Triglycerides are fats derived both from the fatty foods in our diet and from the conversion of excess carbohydrates and proteins into glucose which is converted into saturated fat.)

4. An LDL cholesterol level above 130 mg/dL. The *ideal* value for this lipid is under 100 mg/dL.

5. A fibrinogen level above 350 mg/dL. (Fibrinogen forms clots -- a value of 200 - 250 mg/dL is ideal.)

6. An increased degree of platelet stickiness. Such stickiness can cause clots to form.

7. Elevated levels of homocysteine. (see next page).

These people need the following three *additional strategies:*

1. Take Antioxidant and Homocysteine-Lowering Vitamins

"Free radical" is a popular term used to explain nearly everything that goes wrong in the body from cancer to heart disease and from arthritis to cataracts. This term refers to oxygen atoms which have lost electrons. These electron-deficient (oxidized) atoms severely damage neighboring atoms by robbing them of their electrons.

Current theory suggests that only oxidized low-density lipoprotein cholesterol (LDL) damages the arterial wall. If further studies show this to be true, determination of LDL levels will be important in the prediction of an individual's risk of developing a heart attack.

Chemicals that prevent free radicals from doing damage are called "antioxidants." Of foods with such properties (as fruits, vegetables, legumes, nuts, and seeds), blueberries have the most. In addition to enjoying a healthy, nutritious diet, protect yourself further against these "radicals" by taking 50 mg of vitamin B6, 500 mg of vitamin C, and 400 units of vitamin E daily. These vitamins only cost about 20 cents a day. Further, we suggest that people with multiple risk factors also take 30 mg of coenzyme Q-10 daily. This powerful antioxidant costs about 50 cents a day.

We also suggest that you take a multivitamin that has 0.4 mg of folic acid and 10 mcg of vitamin B12 daily. These vitamins along with vitamin B6 reduce the blood level of *homocysteine,* an amino acid, which in high concentration (above 12 micromols/L) injures endothelial cells and predisposes the inner arterial wall to the development of atherosclerosis. Smoking, inactivity, and dietary factors that cause atherosclerosis also increase homocysteine.

2. Reduce the Stickiness of Your Platelets if They Are Too Sticky

The degree of stickiness that platelets can develop is unique to each person. Platelets that become *very sticky* can cause fatal blood clots. Such platelets may *adhere, activate,* and *aggregate* on the diseased flow surface of atherosclerotic arteries, especially when soft plaques rupture and release their deadly lipid contents into the blood. These platelet aggregates may cause clots to form which can block the channel and stop the flow of blood to vital regions. Such lack of blood supply causes heart attacks, strokes, high blood pressure, blindness, kidney failure, decreased walking capacity, and ulcers and gangrene of the feet and lower legs.

Life depends on an almost endless series of checks and balances of which the stickiness of our platelets is but one example. If our platelets couldn't stick together, we would *bleed to death.* But if they are too sticky, we would *clot to death.* What we want is the right balance.

Millions of people take an aspirin a day to reduce the stickiness of their platelets even though they don't know whether this is either necessary or effective for them. Studies at **The Hope Heart Institute** in Seattle, Washington, have shown that about 25% of people don't need aspirin because their platelets aren't sticky. The other 75% of people have sticky platelets. About 2/3 of these sticky platelet people have platelets that respond adequately to aspirin and 1/3 do not.

The only way to find out who needs treatment to control excessive platelet aggregation and with what medication is to *do relevant tests.* **The Institute**'s staff has developed such tests plus a new medication which works better than aspirin.

3. Select a Good Doctor and Follow His or Her Advice

If your physician finds that you have a "cholesterol" gene problem (such as a very high blood level of LDL with a family or personal history of heart disease at age of 35 to 40 years), he or she may advise the Pritikin or the Ornish diet for you (see p. vi). These diets limit calories from all types of fat to not over 10% of the total (see p. 19 for our preference).

If you retain fluid, your physician will request that you restrict your salt intake. This may also be necessary if you have high blood pressure. It's easy to take too much salt since about 90% of the salt we ingest is already in the packaged, canned, and fast foods we eat. Please read the labels.

Your physician may find that you need medications to decrease your blood pressure, lower your blood levels of LDL cholesterol, triglycerides, glucose, and homocysteine, and raise your blood levels of HDL cholesterol and omega-3 fatty acids. The highest sources of these essential fatty acids are flaxseed and fish oils (pp. 24, 40, 82, 83).

You may need *magnesium* since most people are deficient in this essential mineral that steadies and strengthens the heart beat and decreases high blood pressure.

If you are a woman who has passed through menopause, your physician may advise you to take estrogen or other drugs to reduce your risk of developing osteoporosis, possibly coronary heart disease, and even alzheimer's disease, as well.

While medications are *not* a substitute for the five cardinal rules and the three additional strategies for healthy, fit living, they can be a very important addition when needed.

Appendix

Adipocytes - Cells in the adipose tissue that store fat. The size of these "fat" cells varies directly with the amount of fat they store (Fig. 3, p.5). There are about 100 billion adipocytes in the body. In a very obese person these large, distended cells store hundreds of pounds of fat.

Adipose Tissue - Connective tissue in which the cells, the adipocytes, store droplets of fat that distend them. Adipose tissue was once thought to be largely inert. Now it is known to be very active. Its cells, the adipocytes, synthesize fat from both fatty acids and extra glucose. When glucose is not available to supply calories, the stored fat is released from the adipocytes as fatty acids and used to produce energy. This dynamic process (p. 85) is highly responsive to hormonal and nervous stimulation.

All animals feed intermittently but consume energy continuously, though at varying rates, depending on each animal's physiologic state and degree of activity. Man is no exception. To have energy available for their needs, people must have a means to store fuel. We can store a little less than a pound of glucose as glycogen (1/3 in the liver and 2/3 in muscles), but we can store virtually unlimited amounts of fat (lipids) in the adipocytes of the adipose tissue. Lipids are well suited for this storage because they occupy a smaller volume per calorie of stored chemical energy (9 calories/gram) than either carbohydrates or proteins (4 calories/gram).

The fat content of normal-weight men is about 15-20% of their body weight (Fig. 5, p.8), and for healthy women, about 20-25%. This fat, which is stored in the expandable and contractible adipocytes (Fig. 3, p. 5), represents a 40-60 day supply of reserve energy. In very obese people (Fig. 1, p. 1), their huge fat stores may represent over a year's supply of energy.

Atherosclerosis (Hardening of the Arteries/Arteriosclerosis) - Disease of epidemic proportions in developed nations, where it causes more deaths than all types of cancer, accidents, and infections combined. It is due in large measure to smoking; obtaining too many calories from low-fiber carbohydrates, refined sugar, saturated fats, and *trans* fatty acids; leading a sedentary lifestyle; gaining excess weight (excess stored fat); and letting stress control and distort our lives.

In most patients, this disease causes the inner portion of the arterial wall to become thick, inelastic, and hardened due to plaques formed by infiltration of LDL cholesterol, other fats, and variable amounts of calcium from the blood. Plaques with lots of calcification are hard and those with little are soft. Many soft plaques develop a central collection (core) of thick, slimy, fatty fluid that is covered over by a thin cap of fibrous tissue. If the cap ruptures, this deadly, syrupy liquid in the core oozes inward into the blood where it may trigger the platelets to stick together (aggregate) and cause a clot to form. Such clots are the most common cause of heart attacks.

Atherosclerosis often causes the arterial flow surface to become rough, ulcerated, and depleted of its delicate lining of endothelial cells. Under these conditions, if the blood flow slows or becomes turbulent, the diseased flow surface may cause clots to form which block the channel and stop the flow of blood. Whether by this process or by rupture of a soft plaque with a lipid core, the flow channel can become blocked by clot and cause heart attacks, strokes, decreased walking capacity, limb loss, high blood pressure (hypertension), kidney failure, and congestive heart failure.

In a smaller number of patients, the atherosclerotic process weakens the arterial wall so much, most commonly of the aorta in the mid-abdomen, that the blood pressure forces the wall to bulge out and form enlargements, called aneurysms, which may rupture and cause fatal hemorrhage.

There is a current suspicion, still unproven, that the bacterium, *Chlamydia pneumoniae,* as well as some viruses, may infect the arterial wall and be part of the "hardened" artery problem. The question of which comes first, like the chicken or the egg, will be the subject of much future research.

Body-Mass Index (BMI) - A relative measure of the combined amounts of fat and muscle in the body. This index, calculated by $\frac{weight\ in\ lbs\ x\ 703}{height\ in\ inches\ 2}$, enables degrees of fatness to be compared among different people.

Carbohydrates (plant foods - also see Fiber, pp. 83,84,86) - Organic compounds constructed of carbon, hydrogen, and oxygen, usually in a ratio of 1:2:1. Most of these compounds are polysaccharides which are digested into monosaccharides (simple sugars), mainly glucose ($C_6H_{12}O_6$) and its isomers, fructose and galactose, which are processed by the liver into glucose. Whether glucose is absorbed directly from the bowel or produced in the liver, it is carried by the blood to the cells and used for energy. Also, the body can make any carbohydrate, except Vitamin C (ascorbic acid) from glucose. *Sucrose* ($C_{12}H_{22}O_{11}$) -- *table sugar,* processed from sugar cane and sugar beets -- is a non-fiber disaccharide which is quickly broken down into glucose and fructose by the addition of water. The cells of the brain and the retina can only use glucose; other cells can also use fatty acids. In starvation, the brain and eye cells become able to use fat, too.

Excess glucose in plants and animals is stored in the same form $(C_6H_{10}O_5)x$, called *starch* in plants and *glycogen* in animals. *Insulin, a hormone secreted by the pancreas in response to increased levels of glucose in the blood, enables the cells to use glucose for energy and converts the excess glucose into glycogen,* which is stored 1/3 in the liver and 2/3 in muscles. However, a little less than a pound of glycogen can be stored in these sites. Above this limited storage amount, insulin rapidly converts glucose into fat which is stored in the fat cells of the adipose tissue throughout the body. *High levels of insulin block the use of fat for energy.* When glucose levels fall due to fasting or exercise, a rise in *glucagon,* a hormone secreted by the alpha cells of the islets of the pancreas, converts glycogen back into glucose. When all the glycogen is used up, blood glucose falls; insulin levels decrease. This allows fat to be used for energy.

Cholesterol - A fat-like substance $(C_{25}H_{47}OH)$ used by the body in making the retaining walls of all cells, the male and female sex hormones, and the hormones secreted by the outer part (the cortex) of the adrenal gland which controls vital chemistry of stress, minerals, sugar, and water.

Cholesterol is transported in the blood in one of three forms: high density lipoprotein cholesterol (HDL), low density lipoprotein cholesterol (LDL), and very low density lipoprotein cholesterol (VLDL). The high concentrations of LDL, low concentrations of HDL, and high levels of triglycerides which are found in VLDL all predispose to the development of atherosclerosis. VLDL and LDL favor atherosclerosis by increasing delivery of cholesterol into the inner portion of the arterial wall. HDL protects against atherosclerosis by transporting LDL cholesterol in the blood to the liver, which excretes it in the bile. This chemical action decreases the amount of LDL both in the blood and in the arterial wall.

Saturated fats and *trans* fatty acids raise LDL cholesterol levels in the blood primarily because they block the receptors for LDL in the *liver* and other cells. *Excesses* of carbs and proteins also raise LDL levels because they are converted into glucose and then into sat. fat which blocks more receptors.

In general, LDL cholesterol begins to infiltrate the inner wall of our arteries when it rises above 130 mg/dL in the blood, unless the HDL is also high. This is the reason why it's so important to keep our weight under control and not allow the calories from saturated fats and *trans* fatty acids in our diet to exceed 10% of the total calories we consume in a day. Calorie wise, a little fat goes a long way. LDL cholesterol is bad only if it gets too high. It's a little like water - - we can die of dehydration if we don't have enough, but we can drown in it if we have too much. We need the right amount. LDL cholesterol below 100 mg/dL is best.

Coronary Heart Disease Due to Atherosclerosis - A condition in which the walls of the coronary arteries become thick and hardened due to atherosclerosis (pp. 78, 79). People with coronary disease often experience pain in the left side of the front of their chest during exercise or emotional stress. If you have this symptom (angina), see or call your doctor promptly.

The blood channel of diseased coronary arteries may close off completely from clot formation (p. 79). The heart muscle, deprived of its circulation, may die due to lack of oxygen and nutrients. This is a "heart attack" (p. 84).

Diabetes - A condition characterized by thirst, fatigue, high blood sugar, increased output of urine, and inability of the cells to use glucose due to lack of, or insensitivity to, insulin, a hormone secreted by the beta cells of the islets of the pancreas. Diabetes is the most common cause of blindness and kidney failure, and predisposes to hypertension and atheroslcerosis.

There are two types of diabetes, type 1 (juvenile) and type 2 (adult-onset). Of the 16 million diabetics in the U.S., one million are type 1, and 15 million are type 2. Type 1 diabetes occurs most often around puberty. Many researchers believe that this type of diabetes is due to a viral infection which causes lymphocytes of the immune system to destroy the beta cells of the pancreatic islets. When this happens, the pancreas can't make insulin and the individual must then receive daily injections of this hormone for life. But new research suggests that islet transplants may work for these people.

Type 2 diabetes occurs most frequently in middle-aged, obese adults. But this type is being seen with increasing frequency in younger, obese adults and even in obese children. For unknown reasons, many fat people become resistant to insulin. To compensate, the pancreas secretes more insulin. This works until the exhausted islet cells cannot secrete enough insulin. The initial (and often successful) treatment of type 2 diabetes consists of a diet and exercise program to lose excess fat and add muscle. If such a program isn't adequate, insulin injections and/or oral medications to stimulate the pancreas to secrete more insulin will be necessary. *Prevention is better.*

Emphysema - A condition mainly caused by cigarette smoking which destroys the elastic tissue of the lungs and slowly suffocates the individual.

Fats (Triglycerides) - Molecules that consist of three fatty acids chemically linked to a three-carbon chain alcohol called glycerol. Fats contain mixtures of different types of fatty acids. These acids consist of linear chains of carbon atoms with hydrogen atoms bound to them. Ninety-five percent of the fat stored in the fat cells of the adipose tissue is in the triglyceride form. The adipose cells have a huge capacity to store fat (Figs. 3 & 7, pp. 5 & 11).

Fats may be classified as saturated or unsaturated. A saturated fatty acid has no double carbon=carbon bonds; all of the available bonding sites are filled with hydrogen atoms. Unsaturated fatty acids contain one or more double carbon=carbon bonds. If a fatty acid has only one double bond, it is called monounsaturated. If it has two or more, it is called polyunsaturated.

Saturated fats, except for coconut and palm oil types, are solids at room temperature, while unsaturated fats (oils) are liquid. Both varieties are insoluble in water. The body uses many fatty acids and can make all but two, alpha linolenic and linoleic, which are polyunsaturated and must be in our diet. Because of this, they are "essential." Linoleic acid has a double bond between carbons 6 and 7 (omega-6). Alpha linolenic acid has a double bond between carbons 3 and 4 (omega-3). The ideal ratio of omega-6 to omega-3 fatty acids is about 4:1, or even lower. In the average American's diet, the ratio is much higher, being an unfavorable 20:1, or worse (p. 40).

Each fat or oil is a unique combination of fatty acids, including saturated, monounsaturated, and polyunsaturated omega-6 (linoleic) and omega-3 (alpha linolenic) types. Olive (omega-9), canola, avocado, and peanut oils are *mainly* monounsaturated and protect against atherosclerosis. Listed oils ranked in order of their polyunsaturated omega-3 fatty acid contents are:

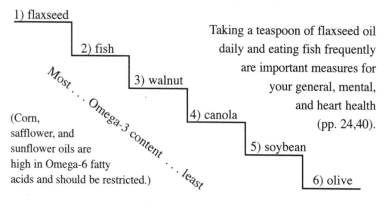

1) flaxseed

2) fish

3) walnut

Most ... Omega-3 content ... least

(Corn, safflower, and sunflower oils are high in Omega-6 fatty acids and should be restricted.)

4) canola

5) soybean

6) olive

Taking a teaspoon of flaxseed oil daily and eating fish frequently are important measures for your general, mental, and heart health (pp. 24,40).

The higher the omega-3 content of an oil, the more it protects against heart disease. Fish (*e.g.,* salmon and tuna) and flaxseed oils are most protective.

Diets high in saturated fats and *trans* fatty acids increase the blood level of low density lipoprotein cholesterol (LDL). When above 130mg/dL, the risk of developing atherosclerosis is elevated. This is so because the saturated fats and *trans* fatty acids reduce the activity of the LDL receptors which are the main mechanism whereby LDL cholesterol is removed from the blood stream by the cells of the body, primarily by those in the liver. Prime sources of saturated fats are whole milk, cream, butter, high-fat cheeses, fatty meats, unskinned poultry (skin has nearly all the fat), candies, many salad dressings, cakes, pies, rich ice creams, and most other desserts.

Hydrogenated or partially hydrogenated vegetable oils (pp. 20, 86, 87) are prime sources of *trans* fatty acids. These include treated soybean and canola oils which are used in the manufacture of margarines, especially the hard types, and products made with margarines, such as many types of cookies, crackers, cakes, candies, chips, dips, doughnuts, pies, and other pastries. Hydrogenation adds hydrogen and converts unsaturated liquid fats (oils) into more saturated solid fats. Beware if the content label reads "hydrogenation" to any degree. Recently, however, the FDA has approved two expensive margarines that have been treated with plant sterols to remove most of the *trans* fatty acids from these products. These new margarines also tend to lower cholesterol to some degree.

Phospholipids, a special type of fat that contains phosphorus, is the main building material for the walls of the 100 trillion cells that make up our body. If these membranes were to dissolve in water, we would die in seconds. From this aspect alone, fat is an essential part of our diet and body. In addition, our brain is 60% fat. But we must be selective in the fats we choose to eat. Saturated fats and *trans* fatty acids can damage our arteries and must be severely restricted because they block receptors and raise LDL.

Many liquid fats (oils) are not only good for us (p. 82) , they add taste and satisfaction to our meals. But oils are such a rich source of calories (9 calories/gram) that they must be eaten in moderation. It's not difficult. Fats and proteins decrease the appetite. Glucose and insulin increase it (p. 22).

Fats are also an important source of energy. If we run for many miles or don't eat for 12 to 18 hours, our main source of energy changes from glucose to fatty acids as our meager stores of glycogen (storage form of glucose) are quickly used up (p. 80). We shift energy gears, so to speak.

Fiber - The portion of plant (carbohydrate) foods that our bodies can't digest. There are two basic types of fiber -- soluble and insoluble. Insoluble fiber (*roughage*) includes the woody parts of plants, such as the skin of fruits and vegetables and the outer coating of grain and rice kernels.

Insoluble fiber helps the digestive system run smoothly and prevents constipation. Soluble fiber dissolves and thickens in water to form gels. Beans, barley, broccoli, citrus fruits, oatmeal, and especially oat bran are rich sources of soluble fiber. Soluble fiber decreases the absorption of cholesterol by the intestines.

Fiber is found only in complex carbohydrates. Whether the fiber is soluble or insoluble, *complex carbohydrates that are protected by an outer covering of fiber are digested and absorbed more slowly than when the fiber has been removed by refining processes.* A high-fiber content slows the digestion of complex carbohydrates and decreases the glucose load on the islet cells of the pancreas. This lowers the demand for insulin and reduces the tendency to develop type 2 diabetes. Fiber also minimizes fluctuations in blood sugar and decreases the appetite. In addition, high-fiber carbohydrates contain many minerals, phytochemicals (plant chemicals), and vitamins. Fiber is indeed valuable.

This is why the majority of our carb calories should come from high-fiber sources, such as fresh fruits; fresh vegetables; legumes; whole-grains (e.g., brown rice, whole wheat, oats, barley, etc., Fig. 9, p. 17); and whole grain breads, cereals, and pastas. **The Better Life Diet** features high-fiber foods.

Low-fiber carbohydrates are digested rapidly into glucose. Because of this, we should *markedly* restrict low-fiber foods, such as white bread, mashed potatoes, french fries (which also have too much fat), and white rice. These carbs and refined sugar cause large quantities of insulin to be secreted.

Heart Attack - A condition in which part of the heart muscle dies because of lack of blood supply, most often from obstruction (occlusion) of a coronary artery due to plaque rupture (pp. 78, 79, 81) and clot formation (thrombosis). The impact of a heart attack may be mild, moderate, severe, or even fatal, depending on how much and which part of the heart muscle has lost its blood supply. The person suffering a heart attack will often experience severe chest pain, become nauseated, sweat profusely, develop marked shortness of breath, have low blood pressure, and feel very weak. The victim may also be seized with chest pain and suddenly "drop dead."

Insulin - A hormone secreted by the beta cells of the islets of the pancreas in response to the level of glucose in the blood. Insulin enables all the cells of the body to use glucose for energy, converts extra glucose into glycogen for storage in the liver and muscles, and stops the use of fat for energy (p. 80). When the glycogen stores are filled, insulin converts any additional glucose into saturated fat which is stored in the cells of the adipose tissue.

Eating habits control insulin production; insulin determines energy source.

As consumption of low-fiber carbs and refined sugars increases, insulin levels rise. When this happens, the body derives more energy from glucose and less from fat.

Consumption	controls	Production	determines	Energy	Source
Low-Fiber Carbs & Refined Sugars	=	Insulin	=	Glucose	Fat
Low-Fiber Carbs & Refined Sugars	=	Insulin	=	Glucose	Fat

As consumption of low-fiber carbs and refined sugars decreases, insulin levels drop. When this happens, the body derives more energy from fat and less from glucose.

Obesity - A condition characterized by storage of excess fat in the adipose tissue, which predisposes the obese person to type 2 diabetes, blindness, kidney failure, hypertension, atherosclerosis, heart attacks, congestive heart failure, strokes, limb loss, cancer, gallstones, and degenerative arthritis.

Osteoporosis - A disorder in which bone structure is absorbed. This weakens the skeleton, shortens its stature, and predisposes the bones to fractures, especially those of the hips and spine.

Platelets - Tiny pinched-off portions of a large bone marrow cell called a *megakaryocyte*. These fragments float along in the outer portion of the blood stream ever ready to initiate formation of a clot to plug up holes in the blood vessel walls. Platelets can also form harmful clots (pp.79,81).

Besides being fundamental in the process of clot formation, platelets release many growth factors that promote the healing of wounds. Platelets survive 10 days after they are released into the blood from the bone marrow. Each second, 1,500,000 platelets wear out and are replaced by 1,500,000 new ones. Too few platelets can cause us to bleed to death; too many can cause us to clot to death. 250,000 platelets/mm^3 of blood is normal.

Proteins - Complex, large molecules constructed of long, three-dimensionally wrapped chains of combinations of amino acids. These acids are molecules constructed of four chemical units joined to a single carbon atom: an amino (NH_2) group, a hydrogen (H) atom, a carboxylic acid (COOH) group, and a side-group containing various combinations of carbon, hydrogen, nitrogen (N), and sometimes sulfur (S) atoms. Side-groups distinguish the 20 different amino acids that our bodies must have.

Of these 20 amino acids, nine can't be manufactured by our bodies and must be derived from our food. These amino acids, which we require but can't produce, are called *essential* amino acids. Our diet must supply them, either from complete or incomplete proteins that are complementary.

The body manufactures thousands of different types of proteins from different combinations of these 20 amino acids. Each of these proteins has a single function which is determined by the order and shape of its amino acid chains. A change of even one atom can impair this vital function.

Many vital structures inside our cells are made from proteins. For example, the ribosomes that make proteins and the mitochondria that generate energy are constructed with proteins. The enzymes that control the chemistry of our bodies are also proteins. The hemoglobin in our red blood cells that carries the oxygen upon which our lives depend is a protein. Our muscles are proteins. The external surface features of our bodies (eyes, ears, nose, skin, hair, and nails) are made of proteins.

Obesity can lead to many serious medical problems. On the other hand, being very thin is also dangerous. If such people can't eat, they must burn more of their already depleted muscles because starving people have no residual glycogen and little remaining fat. Under these conditions, muscle tissue is converted into glucose by a process called "*gluconeogenesis.*" In chronic starvation, death occurs when the body has consumed about half of its muscle tissue for energy (Fig. 7, p.11).

Clearly, proteins are essential for life. And, they provide taste and satisfaction to our meals. Proteins are best obtained from fish, skinless poultry, eggs, legumes (e.g. peas, beans, and lentils in combination with whole grains), nuts, seeds, nonfat/low-fat dairy products, low-saturated fat meat (e.g. lean beef, lamb, and center cut pork loin/chop or roast), and shellfish (e.g. clams, oysters, mussels, crab, shrimp, lobsters, and scallops).

Risk Factors - Conditions that predispose to the development of a certain disease. For example, risk factors for having a heart attack include:
- Smoking.
- Eating a low-fiber diet high in refined sugar, saturated fats, *trans* fatty acids, and calories.

- Leading a sedentary life.
- Carrying significant excess weight (the excess fat in our adipocytes).
- Experiencing marked stress.
- Having a family history of heart disease.
- Possessing dangerous blood findings: sticky platelets, high fibrinogen, low HDL cholesterol, high LDL cholesterol, high triglycerides, high blood sugar (glucose), and/or elevated levels of homocysteine.
- Suffering from atherosclerosis (hardened arteries), hypertension (high blood pressure), diabetes, gout, and/or low thyroid function.

Sugar (Sucrose - $C_{12}H_{22}O_{11,}$ p. 79) - a non-fiber disaccharide (carbohydrate) with a sweet taste. This product (table sugar) is refined in crystalline or powdered form from sugar cane or sugar beets for use in foods to improve taste. Table sugar has only calories -- no fiber, minerals, phytochemicals (plant chemicals), or vitamins. Sucrose is quickly combined with water in the intestines and converted into glucose and its isomer, fructose (both $C_6H_{12}O_6$ monosaccharides). This hydrolytic reaction happens even faster than occurs with low-fiber carbohydrates. Thus, refined sugar should be drastically restricted in our diet because it stimulates insulin secretion which converts excess glucose into fat and prevents its use for energy. Glucose excess, if allowed to progress, will cause obesity with its many serious complications of type 2 diabetes, blindness, kidney failure, hypertension, atherosclerosis, heart attacks, congestive heart failure, strokes, decreased walking capacity, limb loss, gallstones, and degenerative arthritis.

Syndrome X - A condition affecting a growing number of people identified by the chemical triad of low HDL cholesterol, high triglycerides, and a decreased sensitivity of the body's cells to high blood levels of insulin. This triad is associated with a strong tendency to develop obesity, adult-onset (type 2) diabetes, hypertension, and atherosclerosis. The **Better Life Diet and Exercise Program** is well-suited to treat this disorder.

Trans **Fatty Acids (Fats)** - Materials produced by adding hydrogen atoms to the unsaturated carbon chains of vegetable oils. This hydrogenation process changes these oils into materials that are soft solids at room temperature. Examples of such reactions are the conversion of soybean and canola oils in the manufacture of margarines and the conversion of peanut oil in the manufacture of some peanut butters. Because these altered oils contain *trans* fatty acids, they are even more dangerous to your heart than saturated fats. If food labels say "made with hydrogenated or partially hydrogenated oils," avoid these products! Do this because *trans* fatty acids (like saturated fats) block LDL receptors (which are primarily in the liver) and raise LDL cholesterol in the blood.

Index

Special Notes

One day in November, 1999, I had a call from **Thom De Buys,** a very busy Seattle lawyer, who had read my book, *The Open Heart.* He asked me to sign it for him, which I was pleased to do. We started talking, and I was soon very impressed with the magnitude and quality of the dietary information that he had critically reviewed and collected since undergoing urgent quadruple coronary bypass surgery himself in 1995. So, I asked him to critique my nearly finished book, *The Better Life Diet.*

Thom agreed and soon started working with me in an enthusiastic manner to communicate that book's information to the layperson in an even better way. He has continued working with me to make this second edition an increasingly effective means to help people enjoy better health and longer life.

For that immeasurable help, I express my deepest gratitude to him.

Other Books by Lester R. Sauvage, MD
• *The Open Heart: Secret to Happiness* - Forewords by Mother Teresa, MC, and C. Everett Koop, MD, ScD. Dr. Sauvage and ten of his patients tell you from the depths of their souls what matters most in life and how to find it.
• *You Can Beat Heart Disease: Prevention and Treatment* - endorsed by 50 of the world's leading medical authorities. As Dr. David Robinson of the National Institutes of Health said: "All Americans should read this book."

website: www.drsauvage.com

For further information call Better Life Press at 206/323-0116, or visit . . . http://www.drsauvage.com. If you are a book retailer or other book seller, please contact **Independent Publishers Group**, 814 N. Franklin Street, Chicago, Illinois, U.S.A. 60610. Phone: 800/888-4741 or 312/337-0747.